Detox for Life *is a very thorough, entertaining, and informative book on intestinal health. It should be read by all who are interested in preventing cancer and other long-term consequences of bowel toxicity. In caring for cancer patients using multiple modalities over the last 30 years, I have found that detoxification is an indispensable part of the treatment. Many cancer patients have a history of sluggish bowel function throughout their lives, and all have some degree of toxicity.*

— Douglas Brodie, MD, cancer specialist, Reno, Nevada

In a very straightforward and humorous manner, Detox for Life *gets to the heart of vital health: detoxification. As a medical doctor and a proponent of complementary and alternative medicine, I have recommended colon hydrotherapy to those patients requiring it. If you want a comprehensive all-in-one guide to digestive and bowel health for yourself and your family, this book is a must read.*

— Paul Flashner, MD, Wellesley, Massachusetts

Colon therapy is not as American as hot dogs and apple pie, but it will do wonders for your health and life. The waste that exists in your poor, sick body can best be described as cancer that hasn't happened yet. This is a must read! Share it with everyone you care about.

— John Thomas, author of *Young Again! How to Reverse the Aging Process*

Ms. Jordan has put together all the vital information necessary for detoxification in this era of environmental pollution. I congratulate her on a job well done!

— W. John Diamond, MD, co-author of *The Alternative Medicine Definitive Guide to Cancer*

Detox for Life *is a powerhouse of information for anyone desirous of implementing their own tools and strategies for improved health. The guidance it provides can be easily integrated and incorporated into your daily routine.*

— Arthur E. Brawer, MD, Director of Rheumatology Monmouth Medical Center, Long Branch, New Jersey

Detox for Life *is the most thorough book on colon cleansing I have ever seen. It gives excellent understanding about the importance of detoxification, proper digestion, and elimination, and is also an excellent manual for health care practitioners.*

— Pamela Whitney, ND, Smithfield, Rhode Island

Detox for Life *gives careful consideration to the balance of convenience, safety, and efficacy required for success in detoxification. This book is essential for anyone considering holistic cleansing.*

— Mark Pederson, author of *Nutritional Herbology*

From the beginner to the pro, this book offers a motivating, entertaining, and informative look at detoxification and its beneficial effect on overall health. I highly recommend it to anyone interested in decreasing the cumulative effects of aging and its consequences.

— Diane Thorson, DC, BSN

Superb! Detox for Life *is well laid out, very user friendly, and as informative as it could be. Ms. Jordan's concepts are easy to follow and essentially empirical for the cleansing and detoxification of the putrefied colon—the root of numerous diseases!*

— Sharda Sharma, MD, Millburn, New Jersey

I have never known Loree Taylor Jordan to be less than passionate about detoxification, while maintaining a healthy sense of humor about it. This book takes you through the entire process, from the basics of digestion to how to detoxify the whole body, in a very easy-to-understand format.

— L. Pataki, Ph.D., Cs.C.

This is a book of timely urgency. Colon cancer is in the public forefront, and people are becoming increasingly aware of this not-too-talked-about issue. Loree's expertise and outrageous sense of humor will quickly grab your attention with the reality of how a healthy colon can save your life.

— Tom Johnson, Program Director
KEST Radio, San Francisco

Jordan's book gets to the point with detailed information on everything you would ever want to know about colonic therapy, colon health, parasites, diseases, and much more, which she lightens through humor. She relates the information openly and honestly through many of her own personal experiences.

— San Jose City Times

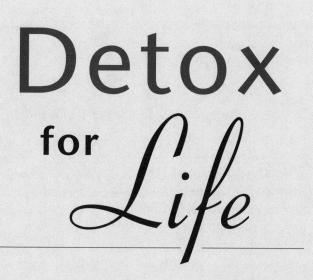

Detox
for *Life*

**Your Bottom Line—It's Your
Colon or Your Life!**

Loree Taylor Jordan, C.C.H., I.D.

Madison Publishing
Campbell, California

Detox for Life © 2002 by Loree Taylor Jordan

Madison Publishing
P.O. Box 231
Campbell, CA 95009
(408) 379-6534

Second printing 2003
Printed in the USA
Illustrations by Steve Ferchaud

ISBN 0-9679878-6-5
Library of Congress Control Number: 2001 129181

The information in this book is for educational purposes only and should not be used to diagnose or treat diseases. If you have a serious health challenge you should consult a competent health practitioner or doctor. It is your responsibility and privilege to gain knowledge and wisdom about your own body so that you may enjoy optimal health. Educational materials produced by the author's company, LTJ Associates, are an independent effort.

Contents

Dedication

Mom, I dedicate this book to you. I can honestly say that if you were here with me, you would read this book and you would laugh your butt off. I know you would be proud of me.

I apologize for not becoming a beautician as promised but ... a colon hydrotherapist? And being crowned "The Colonic Queen"? Do you know how much joke mileage I can get out of my profession? I know that I make people laugh with all this "poop" stuff. But the truth is I know I am saving lives, Mom. Sure, I could give someone a really great haircut or an awesome perm, but so what? It's not an enduring, life-promoting event.

Thanks, Mom, for what you taught me about life in our short 18 years together. I am also grateful that I inherited your outrageous sense of humor—it has pulled me through some tough times. And Mom, even though I can't see you in person, I can see your beautiful smile every day—when I look in the mirror and see my own.

I miss you so much and I love you dearly.

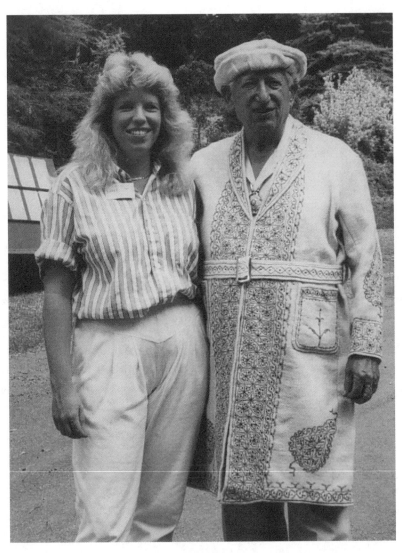

Loree and the late Dr. Bernard Jensen, DC, Ph.D., at his Escondido, California, ranch in 1987. Dr. Jensen is wearing the custom dress of the Hunza tribespeople. Loree is wearing the outdated Farrah Fawcett (yikes) hairdo!

A Special Mentor

I have to say this from my heart: this book would not have been possible if not for the wisdom of one man—Dr. Bernard Jensen, DC, Ph.D. He is truly one of the greatest teachers of all time on the subjects of colon cleansing, iridology, and nutrition. As far as I am concerned, he lives up to his reputation as the father of iridology.

I wrote Dr. Jensen for permission to use some of his charts (which you will see in this book), to thank him for his incredible wisdom, and to express my gratitude for what he taught me. I was told by one of his staff, Lynda, that she would forward my letter to Dr. Jensen, but not to get my hopes up because he did not deal with authors anymore. He happened to come into the office (he was quite elderly now and his office visits were infrequent) and Lynda gave him my letter. He read my letter and graciously gave me permission to use the requested charts. He also sent his best wishes in my endeavors with this book.

Shortly after giving me his blessings, Dr. Jensen passed away quietly February 22, 2001 at his home. I can say wholeheartedly that anyone acquainted with this outstanding man and his teachings will miss him dearly, as I will.

Acknowledgments

If I were to thank everyone who contributed either directly or indirectly to this book, it would sound like an acceptance speech for an Academy Award. I have had the unwavering support of my Dream Team, and you all know who you are. You believed in me, supported me, and carried me when I felt like I couldn't go another step or type another word. Most of all, you made me laugh so I didn't take everything so seriously.

I especially want to thank the health professionals who contributed their voices to this book in the important area of detoxification: Dr. David Ramsey, DC, Director of the New Life Health Center; Robert D. Irons, BS, (son of world-renowned V. Earl Irons); the late Dr. Robert Charm, MD, gastroenterologist, John Muir Medical Center, Walnut Creek, California; and the late Dr. Sebastian Reyes, L.Ac., Doctor of Oriental Medicine.

I would also like to give my appreciation to Morton Walker, DPM, who gave me permission to use the testimonials in his article *The Medical Journalist Report of Innovative Biologics: The Value of Colon Hydrotherapy Verified by Medical Professionals Prescribing It.*

I also want to thank my sons, Brandon and Christopher, who through the years have pushed me to places that I never thought I could go. And I want to acknowledge Brigadoon (a.k.a. Boo-Boo dog) and Ms. Wookie, my dogs and best friends; and Rocky Kitty, who kept me company at my feet on those long marathon writing days.

You are all, truly, the wind beneath my wings.

Foreword

It gives me great pleasure to write the foreword for a book that sheds some light into a dark place: the colon.

Colon health in America is deteriorating. As low-fiber, high-fat, "junk" fast foods proliferate, so will irritable bowel syndrome, hemorrhoids, cancer, diverticulosis, diverticulitis, appendicitis, polyps, and inflammatory bowel disease (ulcerative colitis and Chrohn's). Colon hydrotherapy can play an important role in cleansing and relieving colon pain due to barium enema x-rays, sigmoidoscopy, and colonoscopy.

Physicians are slowly and grudgingly beginning to realize that cleansing from "below" is warranted when cleansing from "above" is ineffective. It is not unusual for me to see fecaliths (round, hard, fecal-matter-like rabbit pellets) sitting in diverticula during a colonoscopy, in spite of an otherwise good colon preparation and clean-out. These fecal collections can remain in place for years and add to the chronic "toxic load" that all of us experience in our lives.

Scientists are beginning to realize that many degenerative diseases, such as cancer and arteriosclerosis, are the result of the accumulation of toxins in our vital organs. Gastroenterologists who understand this path, and the physiology of elimination, might like the eponym "gastroenterexitologist." Most diseases are related to poor eating, poor exercising, poor education, and poor "enjoyment" habits. My theory of Health-e-tivity involves daily eating–enjoyment–education. Proper colon management leads to quality longevity.

All doctors and patients would do well to understand when colon hydrotherapy is indicated, and to experience it for themselves if indicated. My suggestion is that you bring this book, or another one like it, when you visit your personal physician. You may need to seek out an alternative physician who is familiar with, and knowledgeable about, detoxification.

To locate an approved colon hydrotherapist in your area, contact the International Association of Colon Hydrotherapy. Congratulations to Ms. Jordan for her enthusiastic and knowledgeable approach to detoxifying the colon.

– Robert M. Charm, MD
Gastroenterology and Internal Medicine,
John Muir Medical Center

Introduction

Let me tell you a story about Alice, a vibrant young woman, age 36, with two teenage daughters. She had one of the most beautiful smiles you have ever seen. One day Alice went to the gynecologist's office with a suspicious lump in her breast. Her doctor said, "You women just get too hysterical over every little lump. It is nothing to worry about," and sent her home. Six months later she returned to her doctor in real pain and very concerned. This time she was hospitalized for surgery. During the surgery it was discovered that she had a malignant cancer of the breast and it had spread to the lymph nodes. She was given a radical mastectomy. She was advised by her doctor to undergo radiation therapy. Her elder daughter had just received her driver's license and drove Alice to her radiation therapy treatments at the local hospital.

These radiation therapy treatments turned a vibrant young woman with a great sense of humor into a weak and depressed soul, her body literally burned from the inside out with radiation. Alice sat in a wheelchair with tears rolling down her cheeks as her elder daughter got Alice's hair ready for her younger daughter's wedding. Seeing her younger daughter get married should have been one of the happiest days of her life, but Alice was barely able to move, let alone celebrate this joyous occasion. Just a few months later, at the age of 39, Alice quietly slipped away in death, her suffering finally ending.

Alice, you see, was my mother.

I was her elder daughter who drove her to the hospital day after day. I felt her pain and agony firsthand as I watched her life being taken away by the cancer and the radiation, a little more each day. When I was a bride, walking down the aisle to meet my husband-to-be, I was smiling, but there was emptiness and an ache in my heart. My mother wasn't there to share my special wedding day. When I brought home each of my baby sons from the hospital, Grandma Alice was not there to meet them.

I could go on and elaborate all the gory details, all the missed moments in my life after losing her, but what is the point? The fact is that *when anyone dies unnecessarily and very young, everyone loses.* Anyone who has experienced a loved one's battle for their life against cancer—or any debilitating disease— knows it is one of the most heartbreaking things that a family might endure. Losing my mom was a life-changing event that has also been a catalyst, fueling the passion for my work as a holistic health educator.

CHAPTER I

■ ■ ■ ■ ■ ■ ■ ■ ■

"What's a nice girl like you doing in a profession like this?"

Growing up I wanted to be a beautician. I guess I got confused and got at the wrong end.

— Loree Taylor Jordan

People always ask me how I got into this line of work: colonics. Here I am, practicing colon therapy and iridology, when all my life I dreamed of becoming a beautician! I had promised my mother — from a very early age when I loved to style hair — that I would become a beautician. I jokingly admit to being confused and ending up at the *wrong* end. But as often happens in response to a life-changing event, we move inwardly and outwardly, finding places we never knew existed. Perms and hair tints were not to be my destiny. The universe had an entirely different *movement* in mind!

When I was in my early 20s I was invited to someone's house for an herb party, which is somewhat like a Tupperware party. There I met a woman who was both an iridologist and herbalist. She was using a penlight and magnifying glass to look into our irises to determine our health. As bizarre as this sounded, I thought, "Okay, I am open to trying new things." When the woman looked into my left iris she immediately asked me if I had ever broken my left arm. I was stunned.

"Yes," I replied sheepishly. She went on to tell me other issues about my body and my health that were quite accurate.

It was weird, but I had no explanation for the accuracy of her review of current and past health conditions in my body. She explained to us that certain markings in the iris indicate to the practitioner certain health conditions the body may be manifesting (see Chapter 18 on iridology). She also described in detail how the body becomes toxic over time, and how and why we need to cleanse our system with herbs.

It was my introduction to herbal bowel cleansing, and I came home very zealous and enthusiastic about bowel cleansing with herbs. My former husband was less than thrilled that we were going on an herbal cleansing program. I share this story of what happened next as an example of what can occur when one goes on a cleansing crusade without knowing what in the world one is doing!

I wanted to be the captain of this bowel cleansing ship, with my husband being the obedient and supportive shipmate. Our provisions were five different bottles of cleansing herbs I had purchased at the party (actually, two bottles would have been sufficient). Some of these herbs induced diarrhea and cramping if taken too vigorously, but I am the kind of person who believes that if one pill is good, two will be better. You can see where this story is going. We were a young married couple on a bowel cleansing program, with one bathroom … not a pretty picture.

My husband and I took two herbs out of each bottle every three to fours hours. I should mention that he took all these herbs at gunpoint and was resisting me all the way. I also put us on a restricted cleansing diet for 10 days. We were allowed to eat only fruit and vegetables to assist the herbs in cleansing our system.

After about eight hours those herbs kicked in. *Whew!* It was a hurricane going off in both our intestines. I remember at one point my husband shoved me out of the way to get to the bathroom first. Can you imagine a man shoving his adorable young wife out of the way, putting his relief first? It had become every man for himself (or woman for herself in my case). This fecal tidal wave was not for the faint-hearted. My cleansing "Titanic" was sinking fast. It made downing a box of ex-lax seem like a Caribbean cruise.

To say my husband was agitated would be a gross under-statement. I remember at one point he was rolling around on the bed, clutching his stomach, groaning, "Oh my God! My stomach hurts so bad, Loree! Why are you making me do this? I think you are trying to kill me!" If we could fast forward about 15 years I might have harbored such intent, but at that point I was young, naive, and still in love (but that is a whole other book).

Okay, I admit I got a little overzealous here, but I still wanted to complete this 10-day cleansing program successfully. My husband acted as if I had sentenced him to jail for life without any possibility for parole. "Give up junk food for 10 days?" Men can be such whiners, really. But reluctantly he agreed to try and stick it out. I cut down the herb amounts to reduce their impact on our daily schedules. Things calmed down and we weren't hitting each other racing to the bathroom.

About six days into the cleansing program I had hopped into our VW to run an errand. When I returned home I parked in the driveway; my husband was out in the front yard working on the lawn. As I got out of the car I felt my right foot bump up against a paper bag lodged halfway under the car seat. I reached down and discovered a bag from the donut shop with the remains of donuts. Since I had not been to the donut shop I quickly walked up to my husband, stuck the bag under his nose, and pompously asked him if the bag belonged to him. "I don't remember donuts being in the list of fruits and vegetables of our cleansing regime," I told him in my drill sergeant voice. In an absolutely pathetic, wimpy panic, he dropped to his knees and begged me to let him off the cleansing regimen. I must admit I probably was a little self-righteous about wanting to direct this cleansing program, but I wanted us to be healthy, darn it. Why couldn't this man see that? I was doing this for his own good. (Note: Is this the part where I talk about being a flaming co-dependent at that point of my life?) "Do what you want," I snorted, and off I went. And believe me, he went off the cleansing program as fast as you could blink your eyes. He later told me he was reprieved from cleansing hell.

A few hours later a friend, Bob, came over unexpectedly to talk with my husband. Bob had known that we were on an herbal cleansing program and that my husband was less than enthusiastic. When he approached us in the front yard where we were working he looked at me, saluted his hand to his brow, and said sarcastically, "Warden, sir [meaning me], I request permission to talk with the prisoner, sir [meaning my husband of course]!" He stood at attention, stuck out his chest, and clicked his heels. I wanted to hit him with my shovel, but we all started laughing. Okay, I was being a little intense about this bowel cleansing, and now it seemed that I was going to sail this ship on my own with no first mate. (Incidentally, I am still in contact with Bob, who has since done several herbal cleanses himself.)

I did complete the 10 days. But I would have served my husband and myself better by being patient and cleansing slowly the first time around. That was my first, and only, cleansing until my late 20s. You know how life sweeps you up. My life was busy with my two sons. The concept of cleansing kind of floated out of my consciousness. I worried more about diaper rash, cloth versus disposable diapers, potty training, and which was the best preschool. Bowel cleansing was worlds away at that point. As fate would have it, I was destined to learn more about the subject of detoxification than I ever would have dreamed.

In my late 20s I was reintroduced to the fascinating and important subject of bowel cleansing. I went to see a massage therapist, Jane, to have her work on my neck. While I was waiting for my appointment, I picked up Dr. Bernard Jensen's book, *Tissue Cleansing Through Bowel Management,* and I saw pictures that changed my life forever: "stuff" that came out of people's colons. I had heard about this black stuff in the colon at the previous herb class, but hearing about it and seeing it were two entirely different things. This was a visual punch that really hit below the belt!

When Jane came out to get me for my massage, I immediately asked her about these long, black, grotesque, snaky-looking things, and how they could exist in someone's colon. Surely I couldn't have that inside of me!

Jane stated very calmly that everyone has a bowel mucous lining and that we need to work hard at getting rid of the old fecal material to obtain vital health. I found the pitch in my voice rising as I assured her that, at the age of 29, I couldn't possibly have that grotesque stuff in my body. I don't know if I was trying harder to convince her or myself. If I were *that* filthy inside, I would surely know it. I went home, but those pictures haunted me; I asked Jane to help me clean out my colon. I had no idea at that time that this would be a year-and-a-half project. Every few months I went on Dr. Bernard Jensen's 7-day tissue cleansing fast and did a home colonic twice a day, every day, during the cleanse. To some this may sound very radical. But look at it this way—it took years to build up that muck, and it would take some major work to get rid of it.

During this time I was working in the dental field. It was not my passion, but it paid the bills. In 1983, a skiing accident sent me to physical therapy with a full leg cast on my right leg. I got to know my physical therapist, Bill, very well and became very interested in body mechanics, anatomy, the skeletal and muscular systems, etc. I learned a lot from Bill (we are still friends to this day) while healing from the knee injury. I wanted to study the body from the inside out. I was like a sponge trying to soak up everything I could learn about how the body worked.

At this point, if I had not had small children, I probably would have become a physical therapist or a chiropractor. At one point I even thought of going to a holistic medical school in Washington State to become a naturopathic doctor. I realized the commitment necessary to become a naturopathic physician would take me away from my young children too much, and I was not willing to sacrifice them. When I decided to become a mother I committed to being there for them *for the long haul;* any long-term schooling would have to wait.

Instead, I opted to study massage therapy, which was a relatively short-term time investment. I loved working with people and was a very touchy-feely type of person, so this seemed like the perfect profession. I began going to night school to learn massage therapy after my day job as a dental office manager. My husband was very supportive, taking care of our sons for this short time while I was receiving my training. Little did I know that massage therapy training was going to open the door to many other healing modalities.

While working at the dental office, attending massage school, and completing these 7-day cleansings (yes, you can work while cleansing) I talked continuously to the dental aides about bowel cleansing. They teased me at lunch for drinking my cleansing drink. They dubbed it "pond muck" because of its brownish-green color. I took their teasing with a grain of salt because I was becoming very passionate about what I was learning in massage school and in all my reading about bowel cleansing. I was also quite proud of myself for making a sacrifice (no food for a week) to provide my body with the healing I felt was necessary.

I studied every book ever published on bowel cleansing. My former husband used to joke at parties that most people "sit down to read a good novel, but not my wife; she always has her head buried in *The Care of the Colon.*" It was true. I couldn't get enough. As a matter of fact, at one of these parties my friends thought they would "get my goat" by singing a song they had written about me. Four of my friends got up and sang about "The Colonic Queen"! The song was very clever, and absolutely hysterical. We all had tears in our eyes from laughing so hard. That is the night the Colonic Queen was born. I must say that she is alive and well many years later!

Back at the dental office one of the dental aides said to me: "Loree, you are so into this bowel cleansing stuff, you should make this your profession along with your massage. It is all you talk about." Hmm.

Everyone could tell that dentistry was not my passion. Ten years had been enough. Incidentally, one of the staff of this same dental office came to see me as a colonic client 14 years later. You never know whom you will influence! I have teased many of the collaborative members of this book project that they too might be motivated to attempt Loree's Kick-Butt Bowel Blaster after working on *Detox for Life.* They jokingly agree.

In late 1986, along with my friend and classmate Gloria, I took my board exam from the American Massage Therapy Association, using Bill (my former physical therapist) as my model. Bill was a great friend and support, helping Gloria and me study anatomy for our big AMTA exam. We passed with flying colors and soon graduated as certified massage therapists.

In late 1986, after I graduated from the National Holistic Institute in Berkeley, California, I contacted all the chiropractors in the Santa Clara Valley to see if they had room in their offices to accommodate a massage therapist. Dr. David Ramsey did, and we worked out an agreement in early 1987 to schedule me in his office to provide massage therapy two days a week to his patients. This left me to fill the rest of the days with my own clients (who didn't yet exist) and trust that I could match the income of my secure previous position. I was in the mode of trusting the universe.

I had never worked for myself before, but I was so passionate about holistic health that I just knew I would make it. I would virtually stop people on the street to talk to them about holistic health. I had no solid business plan, just faith up the whazoo. This faith paid off. My first year in business, my income from a 4-day workweek was more than it had been working full-time in the dental field. This gave me many blessings: being able to do what I was truly passionate about; helping people with their health; setting my own, more flexible schedule; having more time with my growing sons; and having as much income as I cared to create. I soon had more clients than I knew what to do with. It is really true what they say: "Do what you love and the money will follow."

During all this career-adjusting, and while still raising kids, I continued to be diligent with my cleansing program. I had come a long way from my first bowel explosion disaster. By the fourth time I completed Dr. Jensen's 7-day cleanse, I had not yet "dropped my lining," and my assumption at this point was that I had been right. I knew I was clean inside.

But keep reading. In the summer of 1987, my herbalist friend Marene and I had the privilege of going to Escondido, California, to attend a week-long seminar on iridology given by Dr. Bernard Jensen at his ranch. It was at this seminar that I decided to incorporate iridology into my practice of helping my clients with their health needs. All we heard about for a solid week was how Dr. Jensen helped facilitate the healing of 300,000 patients through colon cleansing, iridology, and detoxification. This really drove home the point that just taking herbs was not enough. Using water through a Colema board (a home colonic unit) or a professional colonic treatment was essential to help strip away the black, gnarly "stuff."

Talk about motivation! Wow! I was *hyped*. I met a gentleman at Dr. Jensen's ranch named Bud Curtis and told him the story of my supposedly clean colon. He advised me to keep going until I dropped that lining, that it would surely be there. So I went home and decided to keep cleansing, to "go for the gold." Actually, I was going for the black, if you know what I mean. The blacker and gooier, the better. Ha!

As fate would have it, on the fifth day of my fifth 7-day cleanse, I was shocked out of my mind. I went into the bathroom and this big, long, black, rubbery thing that looked like an alien from another planet slipped out of my body. *It was about 2½ feet long!* Honestly, if I had seen eyes looking back at me, I would have had a coronary right on the spot. I called my friend, Marene, and told her my gory news. She suggested that if I released any more "stuff," I should take a picture of it like those in Dr. Jensen's tissue cleansing book.

Was that it? Not even close. The next day I put a colander in the toilet to catch any debris so I could actually see how much material was being released. As embarrassing as this might be to mention, I will tell you the truth. I dropped buckets full of black, snaky, goopy, ropy material for the next two days. I felt as of I was giving birth to an alien child. And yes, I did take pictures of my black lining. The smell was the worst thing I could ever imagine, like a decomposing body. So much for my belief that I had a clean colon! The evidence was more than convincing—believe me.

On Sunday, the seventh day of this cleansing—and after the

delivery of this alien afterbirth-looking thing—I developed a 104-degree temperature and went into a healing crisis (discussed in "The Healing Crisis," Chapter 19). I felt clammy, achy, and yucky. I drank plenty of fluids, did another home colonic, and just hung in there. I was actually happy that my body was doing what it needed to do to heal. The next day, as the crisis took its leave, I felt quite a bit better. The very next day, I went to work at Dr. Ramsey's office feeling great.

When I came into the office Dr. Ramsey immediately came over to me to ask me what I had done to my face because he said I was glowing. *Let me think ... I had great sex with my husband over the weekend? Oops, no, that wasn't it. Oh, I dropped about 15 pounds of crusty, gnarly fecal matter out of my bowel. That was it ... glowing skin from cleansing out the bowel and bloodstream.* I told him I had passed that black lining I was always telling him about. He wanted to see the pictures. So I showed him my alien/poop pictures and we just hooted and howled with laughter. We were laughing and cutting up so much our cheeks were aching.

Two days later when I came in to see patients, Dr. Ramsey handed me a card. The card read: "Congratulations on the delivery of your mucous lining!" One of the office secretaries, Charlotte, had signed it too, saying, "Congratulations. I don't understand this but I should probably lose mine, too!" I thought we would all just die of laughter. It had to be one of the funniest moments of my life.

Throughout this time Dr. Ramsey and I worked as a great team. He provided chiropractic care and nutritional counseling, while I provided massage therapy and iridology analysis of the patients. In all of our work together, the health benefits to our patients was our primary concern.

Then life, as it often does, took a turn, requiring that I move out of the area in the summer of 1989. I moved only 45 minutes away, to Hollister, California, but it was far enough that I decided to leave my practice. Of course this meant starting a new practice, in a new area, all over again. The town of Hollister was to give me a run for my money, and at times I felt that the universal support that had been shining on me had disappeared behind a dark rain cloud.

The massage therapy ordinance for Hollister was designed to discourage prostitution—not legitimate massage therapists. But setting up my practice was turning into a nightmare. I could not set up an office from which to operate because of the strict ordinances. Being the "Norma Rae"–type person I am, I negotiated with the city council, the planning commission, and directly with the mayor himself (I called him at home), and got them to adopt a more appropriate massage therapy ordinance. This was a tedious process and quite frankly a pain in the butt. After much literal wrangling with City Hall I was finally able to set up my practice.

I was determined at this point and pressed on. I would educate those meat-eating and steer-roping cowboys if it was the last thing I did. I even sat on the doorstep of two local newspapers and bugged them without mercy until they allowed me to write a weekly article on holistic health. One column was "Loree's Holistic Viewpoint." The weekly newspaper column went over very well. I was beginning to make a name for myself in Hollister.

Then, as fate would have it, in March of 1991 an arsonist's fire destroyed my building and those of eight other business owners. The fire took out the whole block.

Everything in my business was destroyed. Everything I had worked for was gone in just a few minutes. That was a real blow to my entrepreneurial spirit. But I did as I usually do. I picked myself up and kept going, though not without great challenge and effort at times. The financial strain was great; I had to file a lawsuit to regain my financial footing from the fire loss. The whole episode was very hard on my family and on me.

Through all those upsets I kept seeing my clients (at one point temporarily in the back room of a barbershop) and plugging along, doing what I passionately believed in. At one point someone asked me why I didn't just give up my practice and get a real job. It would have been much easier. True. It might have been easier, but not more satisfying. I wanted to serve people in the capacity that filled my soul. I share this with you to show you how completely committed I am to holistic healing.

After wrangling with the insurance company for 18 months, I was finally compensated for my fire loss and was able to rebuild my business. I located a beautiful corner building in the downtown section of Hollister, that was in reconstruction from the Loma Prieta earthquake, to rebuild my holistic health center and create a health food store. If I do say so myself, Loree's Health Store was a beautiful store and should have become a great asset to Hollister. Alternative and Holistic Therapies (my holistic part of the business) was located upstairs, above the store. This was a landmark historical building, and I decorated and furnished the whole top floor in a Victorian theme. It was beautiful — warm and inviting. The Hollister mayor was so proud of my accomplishment that he used to bring visitors upstairs to show them the beautiful health center I had created.

It felt like the right time to incorporate colon hydrotherapy as a modality in my practice. I had previously referred my clients to other colon therapists or had them do a home colonic with my herbal programs. Now I was able to provide colonics myself. This enabled me to be a more supportive presence for my clients through their cleansing process. I was so excited to have my new colonic equipment. The Colonic Queen now had her beautiful castle.

The town did not patronize my health store as much as I

had hoped. Unfortunately, when the health store pulled a "Titanic," the holistic health center went down with the ship.

The other thing that went down with this fast-sinking ship was my 21-year marriage. In 1995 I filed for divorce. I made the joke of demanding those poop pictures in my divorce settlement. I told my former husband, "Here, you can have all the furniture—just give me the poop pictures." Through many moves they have been misplaced, but so be it. It would take me another 30 years of bad eating to grow enough gunk for new pictures.

With pets and two teenage sons in tow I decided to move back to the Bay Area. Once again I had to start over—not just in my practice, but in my life. The last time I had been on my own was when I was 18 years old with a dying mother. But as you can see, adversity has shown up many times in my life and somehow I managed to pick myself up by the bootstraps and go on.

I restarted my practice in the Bay Area and the rewards have been many. I have known in my soul that I am a teacher and educator. I want to teach others, at whatever their own level of understanding, about holistic health.

In March of 1997 I was a radio guest on KEST 1450 AM on the "Robert Perala Show" to promote my upcoming health seminar in the Bay Area. I got bitten by the radio bug and was approached by the producer to think about hosting and producing my own radio show.

I did not have to think very hard! Two weeks later I was on the air as "The Colonic Queen Live," a one-hour call-in show. This was the perfect arena to inform my listeners about colon health. I decided not to be shy and to just "tell it like it is." I talked about poop! I talked about parasites! We laughed! Listeners were appalled and excited about the information, all at the same time. I developed a loyal radio following. Coming on the air saying I was the "Colonic Queen" and that I was passionate about poop was working. Listeners were pleasantly shocked by my outrageousness, about what goes on in the bathroom, or worse, what comes *out* in the bathroom.

The program director, Tom, came into the studio one morning and said to me, "I was listening to your segment this morning [the subject was parasites] and I was eating my breakfast and, Loree, I had to turn you off. You were making me sick." I just laughed. When the general sales manager, Andrea, told him about all the positive phone calls I had received in response to the parasite show Tom was shocked. "What do I know?" he muttered. Actually the funny responses from the listeners about this gross-subject-that-no-one-talks-about gave me permission to be even more outrageous.

One of my favorite people in the radio studio, and on this planet in general, was a tall, handsome black man named Jim Green. He was my engineer for KEST radio station. As I was doing my shows I could always see him through the glass directing me, playing my advertising spots, and so on. This poor guy would turn green listening to all my gory parasite, poop, and bowel-lining stories. He was a riot. His facial expressions were priceless. I teased him mercilessly on the air when he would react to those bowel segments. I even had the listeners believing that he had left me there alone in the studio because he was so repulsed. "Ladies and gentleman ... Jim Green, my engineer, has just left the building." We would laugh. He was a great sport. He also tried my Loree's Kick-Butt Bowel Blaster. How could he avoid it, hearing me talking week after week about dirty colons?

In the fall of 1999 I made a major decision. The following excerpt from a letter entitled "The Colonic Queen Speaketh" was sent to all my friends and clientele, aptly describing what I was going through.

So many times we are running so fast in our lives to the next appointment, to get the kids to soccer practice, to the next work assignment, etc., that we lose sight of our passions and our dreams. Sometimes in all this we even lose sight of who we are and what gifts we are destined to share with others. Some recent challenging experiences in my life have given me the opportunity to look at my life from a much different perspective. I chose to really look and examine, rather than to see my life rush by me from the car window as I was hurrying to get somewhere. I have really searched my heart and realized that my dreams and passions have been set to the wayside while I have been in full-time practice as a colon hydrotherapist.

Even though I have loved meeting each and every one of you during your colon hydrotherapy treatments, there is a lot of focus needed in running a full-time practice. My dreams of writing my books, creating audiotapes, continuing with my professional speaking career, and taking my radio presence nationwide are calling out so loudly that I must listen. Rather than providing colon therapy services myself, I aspire to write and create materials to educate others on a grander scale. As one friend stated to me, "We have been hearing about your book for three years now, so let's get to it, already." She is right! So I plan to "get to it, already" and not just dream about it.

Actually, my book, DETOX FOR LIFE, will be out soon. It will be the lighter side of colon cleansing. Anything is possible if you dream big enough.

I would like to take this time and opportunity to say thank you for your business and friendship. My wish for you and your families is continued good health and many blessings.

– Loree Taylor Jordan

With that said, in the fall of 1999 I sold my colon hydrotherapy practice so I could concentrate on expanding my message via radio, television, and print to others on a national scale. Once again I was asking the universe to support me in this dream and vision.

After selling my practice I was flying home from a trip to Oregon, and sitting next to a pleasant woman, Ginger, who was more than polite as I crawled over her many times to go to the bathroom. I forgot to tell my travel agent to give me an aisle seat. I am not the person to travel with—I have a bladder the size of a lentil bean.

As we struck up a conversation, we discovered that we had the same middle name—Taylor—and that we lived just a few miles apart. In the course of the conversation I told her I was an author-in-progress, working on my first book. I always hold my breath when people say: "Oh, a book! How wonderful! What is it about?"

Oh boy, here it goes! I answered: "Detoxifying the body through colon hydrotherapy."

"Well that is certainly an unusual topic," she laughed! It turned out that she ran a marketing company and was looking for women speakers for a yearly women's health conference in the Bay Area. She was trying to field a variety of health subjects and mine was definitely unique. So we exchanged phone numbers, information, and so on. Get this: As I write these words she has me scheduled to speak at this year's women's conference; she also has scheduled me as a guest on a Bay Area women's cable TV show to promote my upcoming book! How is that for universal support? I think the universe is doing pretty well right now ... don't you?

CHAPTER 2

■ ■ ■ ■ ■ ■ ■ ■ ■ ■

The Art of Mastication and Digestion

It's often said that you are what you eat. I say that you are what you absorb.

– Bernard Jensen, DC, Ph.D.

MASTICATION

For all the *guys* who turned to this chapter first: this is not what you think it is. You're thinking of the other "M" word. Here, I am referring to chewing. Yes, chewing. You're about to get a private lesson in *mastication.* You might think I'm crazy to try to tell you how to chew your own food, but believe me, it is vitally important. Throughout my years as a colon hydrotherapist I saw an incredible number of clients with whole food particles and other undigested bits of food coming out of their colon during colonic treatments.

Digestion begins in the mouth as we chew, or masticate, our food. Thorough mastication of food is of primary importance to assure that food completely mixes with oral digestive juices, initiating digestion. Get the digestive process off to a good start. Try to stay focused and aware, thoroughly coating your food with the saliva in your mouth. Also, the more you chew, the more slowly you'll eat. You'll feel full sooner, and will be less likely to overeat. I suggest you sit down when you eat, take your time, take deep breaths. Simply put, *masticate your food into a fluid mass before swallowing.* No solid pieces should be allowed to enter the stomach. Chew your food into the tiniest pieces possible. This creates more surface area on which the stomach acids can act. Large, unmasticated pieces of food entering the stomach cause flatulence and distension of the stomach. It takes longer for the stomach to break down large pieces of food and it uses up more enzymes. The simple mechanical act of proper mastication can mean a world of difference to digestion and assimilation.

Today we are in too much of a hurry to enjoy our food. We often just gulp it down as we run from here to there. Part of eating consciously is pacing yourself. I say *eating in the car is absolutely prohibited*. How can you drive, watch the traffic, probably answer the cell phone, and properly masticate your lunch all at the same time? Admit it. You wolf down your food as you avoid the car in front of you, with your mind on twenty other things, the least of which is chewing your food at a leisurely pace to enhance the digestive process.

Overeating, constant snacking, diluting digestive secretions with liquids, and eating complex mixtures of food can all place undue stress on our digestive organs. When you eat too much or too fast, when you don't chew food properly, or when you are experiencing emotional stress, you are more likely to feel the effects of indigestion—the improper digestion of food. Anger, pain, and emotional upset inhibit gastric secretions. I have said jokingly that if *that* were the case I should not have eaten for the whole 21 years I was married. Seriously, hammering out an emotional or stressful situation is best left for another time, such as a visit to your therapist's office, and not while you're trying to eat!

DIGESTION

Your digestive system is like the power plant of a city. The power plant supplies the heat or spark that causes the fuel to ignite. Its furnaces then burn fuel, convert it to energy, and

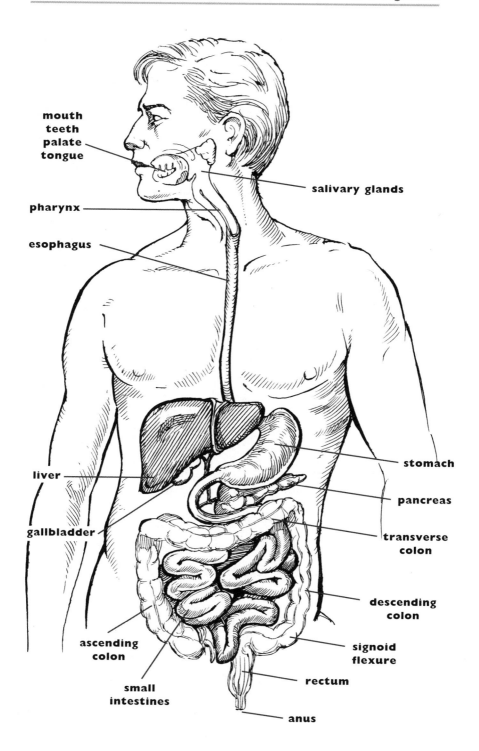

mouth
teeth
palate
tongue

salivary glands

pharynx

esophagus

liver

gallbladder

ascending
colon

small
intestines

stomach

pancreas

transverse
colon

descending
colon

signoid
flexure

rectum

anus

supply the energy to all parts of the city. If the fuel doesn't burn, the city will have no energy. Your body burns fuel to provide the energy needed to maintain your own spark of life—your metabolism. Metabolism may also be defined as the chemical changes that assimilated food undergoes in the cells, for utilization by the body. The body is built, repaired, and fueled by about a half-ton of food per year. This fuel must be selected carefully to provide maximum performance, but just having the right kind of fuel is not sufficient.

The food you eat must be digested and assimilated in order to provide the energy your body requires. The digestive system supplies the spark that initiates the burning (digestion) of your food. If your digestive system is not functioning properly, even the best nutrients will do you little or no good. The various secretions of the digestive system, and most importantly the enzymes, provide the spark to break down your food into energy your body can use.

It's time for a quick tour of the human digestive system. Though it won't take very long, we'll cover 18 million square inches on our journey from the mouth to the rectum (that's 600 times more surface area than the skin). Ready? Take a bite!

Food enters the body via the alimentary canal mucus membrane (which extends from the mouth and throat through the stomach), proceeds through the duodenum, small intestines, the large intestine/colon, and to the rectum for elimination. All along the way the accessory organs, including the tongue, teeth, salivary glands, pancreas, liver, and gallbladder, supply necessary enzymes and key processes that help turn food into energy.

Mechanical, chemical, and physical processes must all work together to accomplish the miracle of digestion. Mechanical processes are accomplished by muscular contractions and rhythmical movements that move the food along the tract at just the right speed so that required chemical changes of the food will occur where and when they are needed.

All living organisms must metabolize food in order to survive. Before the millions of cells in your body can make use of the proteins, carbohydrates, and fats you put into your system, major physical and chemical changes will take place. For example, a chemical change takes place when complex sugars are broken down into simple sugars. A physical change occurs when a solid substance (food) is liquefied. These processes must function efficiently to ensure that the nutrients (potential energy) in the food you eat will be digested, absorbed, and used throughout the body.

The digestion of carbohydrates, for example, begins with a starch-digesting enzyme in saliva. Trivia fact: You produce approximately 3 pints of saliva each day. Starch- and sugar-digesting enzymes secreted by the pancreas and small intestine complete carbohydrate digestion. Carbohydrates are thereby broken down into simple sugars, which your cells can burn for the energy they need to do their respective tasks. Proteins break down into smaller fragments under the influence of hydrochloric acid and pepsin in the stomach. Then they are broken into free amino acids in the intestines by enzymes from the pancreas and intestinal wall. Fat digestion doesn't begin until fats reach the small intestine. Bile salts from the liver and gallbladder make the fats water-soluble so they can be carried through the bloodstream, while enzymes from the pancreas and intestinal wall break the fats into fatty acids and glycerol. When food particle nutrients are small enough, they pass from the small intestine to the bloodstream, where the nutrients are circulated to all body cells. About 90% of absorption of nutrients takes place in the small intestine.

For effective digestion, the stomach, liver, pancreas, gallbladder, and intestines all require food, digestive enzymes, and vitamins to be present, so proteins can hydrolyze into amino acids, and minerals can ionize to form absorbable chelates (provided there are no chelatin-interfering processes present). Problems anywhere along the line can result from an enzyme-poor diet, highly refined foods, pesticides, preservatives, pasteurization, irradiation, food overcooking (104 to 160°F), and from lack of fiber.

ORGANS OF DIGESTION

The *mouth* or *oral cavity*, which links to the pharynx, is composed of the cheeks, the tongue and its muscles (the floor of the mouth), and the hard and soft palates (roof of the mouth). The tongue, the organ of taste, consists of muscles covered with mucus membranes, glands, and taste buds. It assists in chewing, lubricating, swallowing, and digesting. Stimulation to the taste buds on the tongue increases the secretion of saliva and starts the flow of gastric juices. The teeth are extremely important in digestion. Teeth are named according to their shape and use: incisors, canines, premolars or bicuspids, and molars.

In addition to its digestive function, mastication is highly important to oral health due to the massaging effect chewing has upon the gums. The sinking and rising of the teeth in their sockets tends to promote circulation and help prevent gum disease. You need healthy teeth and gums to properly masticate your food. Keep your teeth and gums healthy: thoroughly brush and floss on a daily basis and keep up regular visits to the dentist. I sense my dental training coming back! Oh no! "Once a dental assistant, always a dental assistant."

The *salivary glands* are key players in the art of digestion. Although many minute oral glands pour their secretions into the mouth, the chief salivary juices are supplied by three tiny salivary glands. The salivary gland's secretions are responses to chemical and thought stimulation, and last for 20 minutes after chewing ceases. Starch digestion is initiated by the enzyme protein ptyalin found in these juices.

The *pharynx*, commonly known as the *throat*, transmits foods from the mouth to the *esophagus*. The throat, like the entire digestive tract, is lined with mucous membranes and well-supplied with mucous glands. Food and liquid stimulate and initiate the sensory receptors in the walls of the pharynx and initiate the swallowing reflex. The 10-inch esophagus extends from the pharynx to the stomach and goes through the diaphragm as it enters the abdominal cavity. By wavelike, muscular (peristaltic) contractions, it passes food into the stomach.

The *stomach* is in the upper part of the abdominal cavity, just below the diaphragm. There, the digestive tube dilates into a muscular, pouch-like structure—the stomach. The stomach acts mainly as a reservoir to store food until it can be assimilated in the small intestine. Digestive enzymes from the inner lining of mucous membranes are secreted into the stomach at the sight, smell, thought, or taste of food. About 5,000,000 microscopic glands secrete 1.5 gallons of gastric juices every 24 hours. Along with the gastric juices in the stomach is hydrochloric acid, an indispensable agent in digesting food. But here again, thorough mastication is crucial for hydrochloric acid to work properly.

The upper stomach stores food for an hour or two for predigestion by food enzymes (no enzymes are secreted there) and retains a pH of 6.0. The stomach walls contract to serve a twofold purpose: (1) churning and breaking down food into smaller pieces, and (2) thoroughly mixing food with gastric juices in preparation to assist digestion.

After the stomach has completed its digestive work, the semifluid mass (chyme) enters the *small intestine* through the pyloric valve. The three parts of the small intestine are: (1) the 10-inch duodenum, attached to the lower end of the stomach and resembling the letter "C"; (2) the 8-foot jejunum; and (3) the lower portion, the ileum, which is about 12 feet long. The ileum joins the large intestine at a right angle and under high pressure. The ileocecal valve acts as a guard at this junction to prevent the return of material that has been discharged into the large intestine. In other words, this is a one-way valve. Material going into the large intestine cannot return into the small intestine.

The greatest amount of digestion and absorption occurs in the small intestine, which is especially structured for this purpose. There are approximately 4,500,000 villi, small finger-like projections found in the small intestine, that increase its absorptive surface. The digested food passes into the capillaries and lacteals of the villi, through the lymph system, into the bloodstream, and then on to the cells. Most of the small intestine is arranged in circular folds that provide more surface area for absorption and that lengthen the time of passage of food through it, allowing more thorough action and mixing of food mass with digestive fluids. The numerous glands covering the wall of the small intestine secrete mucus and an alkaline digestive fluid containing enzymes.

THE COLON

The *large intestine*, also known as the *colon*, is 2½ inches wide and has three times the diameter of the small intestine, but measures only 5 feet in length. The colon is a continuous tube, subdivided into three main parts:

1. The *ascending colon* (on the right side of the abdomen), where digested food is still liquid, joined at the ileocecal valve to the small intestine.

2. The *transverse colon*, which runs transverse across the abdomen and under the rib cage. The transverse colon includes the splenic flexure under the left rib cage and the hepatic flexure above the liver, under the right rib cage.

3. The *descending colon* (on the left side of the abdomen) descends down the left side of the body where the food beyond is beginning to solidify. In the large intestine most of the water content and mineral salts are absorbed back into the body. The

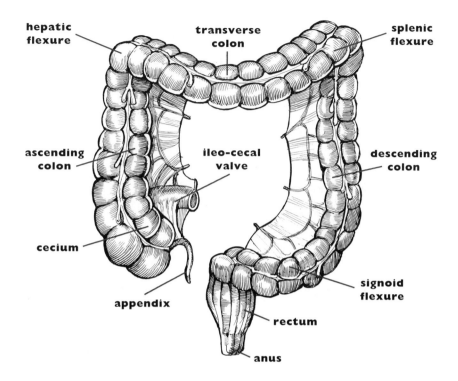

hepatic flexure
transverse colon
splenic flexure
ascending colon
ileo-cecal valve
descending colon
cecium
appendix
signoid flexure
rectum
anus

semisolid waste remaining is still 60 to 70% water, and is also 10 to 30% bacteria, with the remainder being indigestible cellulose material, dead cells, and other waste materials. The smooth muscular walls of the colon contract (peristalsis) to move waste through the colon. This takes anywhere from 12 to 24 hours or longer, depending on the amount of roughage present. Many people have what is called an "atonic bowel," which means that the bowel has lost its peristaltic ability to contract and move waste through. This condition is largely attributable to a lifestyle of heavily refined foods, and a lack of fiber and roughage in the diet. The descending colon adjoins the *sigmoid colon,* an S-shaped curve that stores feces for disposal. I have seen many clients with this part of the colon ballooned out by impacted fecal matter the body is unable to release.

The eliminative mechanism, the *rectum,* makes up the last 7 to 8 inches of the intestinal tube; and the *anus,* or anal canal, the elimination valve, is the terminal inch of the rectum. Principally, the purpose of the colon is to reabsorb water and electrolytes and to solidify feces, but some absorption and digestion also takes place in the ascending and transverse colons. The ascending and transverse colons are digestive areas, while the descending colon, rectum, and anus are storage areas containing limited absorptive area.

ACCESSORY ORGANS OF DIGESTION

The *pancreas* is a soft, pinkish-gray gland that, because it performs both external secretion (on the surface of the pancreas) and internal secretion (into the bloodstream), is known as a compound gland. The pancreatic juices that empty into the small intestine through a common duct contain three essential digestion enzymes: (1) trypsin, which breaks down protein into amino acids; (2) amylase, which acts on carbohydrates, changing compound sugars to simple sugars; and (3) lipase, which reduces fats to fatty acids. If the pancreas is damaged, infected, or worn out, or if there is blockage preventing the pancreatic juice from reaching the intestinal tract, serious digestive and malabsorptive problems may ensue.

The internally secreted hormone insulin, produced by the 20,000 to 1,000,000 microscopic cells known as the Isles of Langerhans, is essential in controlling blood sugar. A person deficient in or lacking this hormone develops diabetes, a disease in which the body cannot utilize carbohydrates.

The 3½- to 5-pound *liver* is not only the largest gland in the body, but may be the most miraculous in its diversity of life-sustaining functions. The liver performs over 500 functions in the body. For our purposes I will refer only to the role the liver plays in digestion. The liver can be felt with the fingers on the right side just below the rib cage.

The numerous and complicated functions of the liver are indispensable in the maintenance, regulation, and homeostasis (state of constancy) of body fluids, and in the control of the body processes. The liver can be compared to a chemical laboratory, storage plant, distribution service, warehouse, power plant, and waste disposal plant, because of its phenomenal assemblage of structures, machinery, and production. Its major functions can be categorized as follows:

1. *Secretory and excretory functions.* The daily secretion of bile (a pint to a quart) is necessary to facilitate fat digestion and absorption, and to excrete certain waste products.

2. *Metabolic functions.* The liver plays an essential role in the metabolism of carbohydrates, proteins, and fats. The metabolic processes concerned with carbohydrates are fundamental to maintaining blood glucose levels. This organ stores glycogen, which has been synthesized from proteins as well as from sugars, and converts glycogen to glucose to maintain blood sugar constancy. Fats are broken down by the liver for utilization by the body. The liver's manufacture of blood proteins is basic to proper body functioning and survival.

3. *Detoxification.* One of the most important roles of the liver is its protective role in detoxifying harmful substances. Through bile, the liver is able to eliminate certain drugs and heavy metals. Through the phagocytic action of the kuppfer cells in the liver, injurious materials such as bacteria and poisons are removed from the blood. If you wanted to build a physical plant that would reproduce materials manufactured by the liver, separate the toxins, purify the various poisons, and perform other liver functions, you'd need a building five stories high and one block square. It would have to feature the ultimate in technology and yet still couldn't perform all the functions of your 5-pound liver.

The *gallbladder* can contract and expand like the stomach. The important secretion bile, composed principally of bile salts, bile pigments, cholesterol, and water, is essential for the absorption of vitamin K and other fat-soluble vitamins. Bile pigments from worn-out blood cells reduce the acidity of the chyme (liquefied food) and give the yellow-brown color to the feces. Bile is necessary to aid digestion of acid foods. The mere presence of acid food in the stomach causes the common duct to open and discharge bile into the small intestine.

So there you have it! After this lesson in digestive anatomy it should be quite clear that your digestive health is absolutely vital to your overall health. All your digestive organs work together in a symphony of digestion. Just as a perfect orchestra has all its instruments playing in harmony to create a beautiful masterpiece, the digestive system too is designed to orchestrate digestion in perfect harmony. Support your local orchestra: take care of your digestive system. It all starts with learning how to masticate!

CHAPTER 3

■ ■ ■ ■ ■ ■ ■ ■ ■ ■

Proper Food Combining

Drum roll, please! You are on the threshold of learning a new way of eating. In the previous chapter you learned *how* to enhance digestion. This chapter deals with *what* and *when* to eat. This is vital information to incorporate into your lifestyle forever. You can start right now to experience the well-being you deserve and that is your birthright. Your body wants to shine. All you have to do is facilitate its natural processes, and you can start to experience the joys of vibrant and vital health.

You must eat food in combinations compatible with your digestive chemistry—this is mandatory for optimum health. Just like anything else, the digestive system has certain limitations. The goal here is to eat food in accordance with the laws of digestion and not work against them, thereby discouraging toxemia (toxic buildup). Digestion requires complete energy and attention from the body. That is why after a large meal (or an improperly combined meal) you feel tired and drowsy. Your body puts all of its energy into digesting the food and does not have energy for anything else.

Many of our most familiar food combinations work against the laws of our digestive nature. I believe that all over-the-counter digestive aids on the market today could be eliminated if people followed the guidelines of proper food combining. People in the United States spend more than $2 billion a year on digestive aids. Gas, bloating, and an upset stomach after eating are the norm these days.

I remember seeing a commercial a few months back that left me with my mouth hanging open. It was a scenario of a couple in their mini-van, with kids in the back seat, at a drive-through restaurant. The gist of the ad was: if the wife took Brand X digestive aid then she could indulge in eating the highly processed foods offered at this fast food restaurant. Unfortunately, it is a fairly accurate depiction of the level of understanding of the general public. Just take a pill for the ill of the moment and the symptoms will go away. Then, to add insult to injury, they scarf down hamburgers and greasy french fries. Sure, that's the solution!

I can tell you that proper food combining and digestive enzyme support relieved about 90% of the digestive problems that plagued my clients. Many clients who had suffered for years were absolutely blown away at the digestive relief they obtained with such a simple lifestyle change as proper food combining. Sometimes I had to use herbs to calm down the digestive fire in the intestinal tract. The mucous membranes were literally burned and raw from gastric juices.

It is important to mention that, even though you don't experience obvious pain after eating an improperly combined or junk food meal, your body is still suffering from digestive abuse. If you violate the laws of digestion and proper food combining, your body *will* suffer. We eat food to nourish our bodies and sustain life. If food is not sufficiently broken down for conversion to usable energy, the body winds up having to dispose of large amounts of waste material. In Chapter 8, "Auto-intoxication," I will go into greater detail about the dangers of creating more waste than the body can handle. It's a disease waiting to happen.

It is really important to understand that two of the most dangerous weapons we can use against ourselves are the knife and fork. I want to help you develop a consciousness about food and what effect it has on your body as a whole. Stanley

Burroughs, author of *The Master Cleanser*, goes as far as to say, "If you have a disease it's because you ate it."

I know these new principles will fly right in the face of the way most of us were brought up around the supper table. The ol' meat and potatoes dinner, rice and fish, eggs and toast, milk and cereal, grilled cheese sandwiches, macaroni and cheese— we've eaten them all.

People usually panic when they first see proper food combinations. *Don't panic.* Once you understand the concepts of food combining you will be able to follow them with ease. Besides, you will have so much energy and you will feel so great that you won't even care that you cannot eat junk food anymore. Trust me, this is a good thing.

NATURAL HYGIENE

Let's take a look at the basic law of natural hygiene as it relates to the body's physiological cycles. Extensive research has been done on physiological cycles, most notably by the Swedish scientist Are Waerland, and by T.C. Fry of the American College of Health Science. These cycles are based on rather obvious functions of the body. To put it in its simplest terms, on a daily basis you take in food (appropriation), you absorb and use some of that food (assimilation), and you get rid of what you don't use (elimination).

Natural Body Cycles

Appropriation (eating & digestion)	12 noon – 8 p.m.
Assimilation (absorption and use)	8 p.m. – 4 a.m.
Elimination (of body waste)	4 a.m. – 12 noon

While the times indicated above might vary slightly due to various factors, your body's cycles are recognizable if you simply observe your body in action.

What Foods Can and Cannot Be Combined Successfully

We define a protein as containing 15% or more protein, and a carbohydrate as containing 20% or more starch.

YES means they are compatible
NO means they should not be combined if you frequently suffer discomfort after meals

YES* with animal fats
NO with vegetable fats

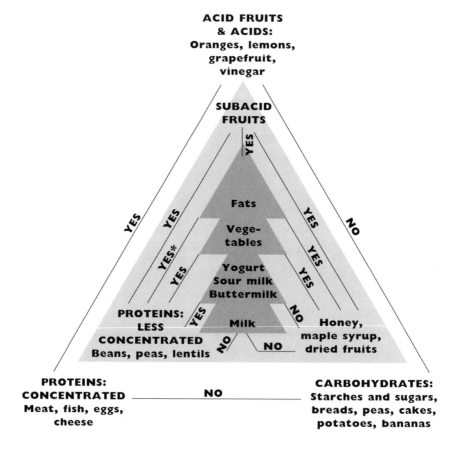

Source: *How to Always Be Well*, Dr. William Hay

BASIC PRINCIPLES OF PROPER FOOD COMBINING

◆ *Eat fruit alone or leave it alone.* It is suggested by the laws of natural hygiene to eat fruit only until noon when the body is in the cleansing and elimination cycle. (See below for special considerations.)

◆ *Eat melons alone.*

◆ *Eat fruit at least* 20 *minutes before a meal* (not after or with a meal). If eaten with a meal, fruit will cause other food to ferment and rot in the stomach.

◆ *Proteins and starches should not be eaten at the same meal.* Proteins and starches cannot be digested efficiently in the stomach at the same time. Protein—including all flesh foods (beef, chicken, fish, pork, or any animal), dairy products, and nuts—demands digestive juices that are acidic in nature. Starches—such as bread, pasta, grain, potatoes (cooked), and cereals—demand digestive juices that are alkaline in nature. Because these digestive juices cancel each other out, the protein and starch if eaten together will just sit and rot and ferment in the stomach.

◆ *Combine proteins with vegetables* at the same meal.

◆ *Combine starches with vegetables* at the same meal.

◆ *Rice and beans can be combined.*

◆ *You may combine 2 starches.*

◆ *You should not combine 2 proteins.*

◆ *Eat one concentrated food at a time* (anything other than a fruit or vegetable is a concentrated food).

Special considerations: Though I am giving a basic overview of a program that contributes to healthy digestion, there are some exceptions. I cannot overemphasize the importance of considering an alkalizing diet for disease prevention. However, one factor may require special consideration when one is on this program: issues with an insulin or blood sugar imbalance. For some, having all that concentrated sugar in the fruit may not benefit their body chemistry. Having an alkalizing breakfast of steamed vegetables might be a better choice.

I personally watch my sugar intake and use an alkalizing green drink in the mornings, and lots of pure water before my workouts. If I want something more, I will have vegetables. I have been known to have a healthy salad for breakfast. I have to really watch my intake of fruit. You and you alone are responsible for your body and how it functions. Make the choice that best serves you and your personal body chemistry. You may want to consult with your health care practitioner for dietary suggestions that are relevant to your needs.

Remember, keep it simple. Your body is 70% water. To maintain your vitality you must consume food that is at least 70% water content. Eat simple, balanced, harmonious meals. Begin your meals with fresh fruit (at least 20 minutes before eating other foods) and vegetables. The purpose of intelligent food combining is to deliver the goods of a balanced diet.

Right food combinations make for more complete digestion, more complete assimilation, and harmonious digestive music. Your body is always striving toward health. Do yourself a favor and get out of your own way. Give your body a chance to function at its highest level, to live with abundant energy—the true essence of life. You know life's gift to you is your body. Your gift in return is to take the best care of it that you can.

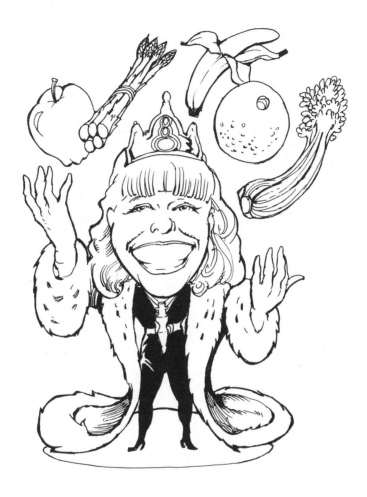

How long should you wait after eating other food before you can again eat fruit?

Salad or raw vegetables	2 hours
Properly combined meal, without flesh	3 hours
Properly combined meal, with flesh	4 hours
Any improperly combined meal	8 hours

CHAPTER 4

■ ■ ■ ■ ■ ■ ■ ■ ■

Food for Thought

Choose a healthy relationship with your diet.
Take full responsibility for everything
you choose to eat, and eat foods
in the spirit of healing consciousness.

Mental clarity and detoxification are also critical in the healing process. Cleansing our minds of negative thought patterns is essential to optimal health. Just as environmental toxins can invade our bodies, negative thoughts, emotions, and stress can increase biochemical toxicity. My gifts to you are positive affirmations to set the stage for conscious choices.

Strive to:

- ◆ Eat your food in the spirit of moderation.

- ◆ Commit yourself to eating nutritionally superior food.

- ◆ Relax before you eat each meal.

- ◆ Remember, good posture counts.

- ◆ Choose and create a healing environment and loving setting for your meals.

- ◆ Plan to eat your meals at regular times during the day.

- ◆ Allow yourself 30 minutes to sit down, and stay totally committed to your meal.

- ◆ Know when enough is enough.

- ◆ Know when not to eat.

- Cultivate a desire-less food consciousness.

- Appreciate the food you eat.

- Approach each meal as you would the breaking of a long juice fast, with enthusiasm, patience, calmness, control, and composure.

- Eat in the healing consciousness.

- Chew your food one bite at a time.

- Chew your food slowly.

- Make your mouth and your teeth your own juicer.

- See that variety in what you eat makes your diet more interesting.

- Enjoy your food and be creative. Take time to enjoy preparing and eating your meals.

- Realize that intimate conversation, good company, and laughter aid your digestion and assimilation.

- Maintain a steady, even, relaxed pace when you eat.

And avoid:

- Overeating.

- Becoming a victim of nervous eating habits.

- Eating when emotionally upset, anxious, uptight, or depressed.

- Constantly snacking, nibbling, tasting, or raiding.

- Consuming harmful foods.

- Eating food containing toxic chemicals or other pollutants.

- Eating food that is lifeless and/or overcooked.

- Consuming more than one-third of your protein in the form of animal protein.

- Becoming emotionally attached to your food.

- Binges—especially with cheese, crackers, ice cream, desserts, fruit, mints, nuts, peanut butter, and dried fruits.

- Overindulging in any one food group or food item.

- Taking your diet for granted.

- Drinking with your meals.

- Mixing fruits and vegetables.

FOOD RESPONSIBILITY

You choose:

- A healthy, emotional relationship with your diet.

- To take full responsibility for everything you choose to eat.

- To evaluate your own diet.

- Foods in the spirit of the healing consciousness.

- Foods on the basis of quality.

- Fresh, living foods (vs. dead, lifeless foods).

- Whole, unprocessed foods (vs. fragmented, processed foods).

- Pure (vs. chemically toxic) foods.

- Natural (vs. synthetically altered) foods.

- Organic (vs. chemically fertilized) foods.

- Raw (vs. cooked) foods.

Commit yourself to:

- ◆ Pure, living, fresh fruits.

- ◆ Pure, living, fresh raw vegetables.

- ◆ Whole grains and whole grain cereals.

- ◆ Whole nuts, seeds, and nut butters.

- ◆ High-quality protein.

- ◆ High-quality fats.

- ◆ High-quality carbohydrates.

Let go of:

- ◆ Refined carbohydrates and refined table sugars (chocolate, candy, ice cream, rich dessert, cake, donuts, white sugar, white rice, and white bread).

- ◆ Canned, packaged, frozen, and processed foods.

- ◆ Salt in or on your food.

- ◆ Hydrogenated cooking oils and refined oils.

- ◆ Hydrogenated fats.

- ◆ Hydrogenated nut butters (purchase in the health food store only).

- ◆ Red meat and its equivalent.

- ◆ Greasy, fried, fatty foods.

- ◆ Excess protein, excess fat, excess starch.

- ◆ High-fat milk, pasteurized.

- ◆ Dead/devitalized foods.

- ◆ Chemically toxic foods.

- Caffeine, instant coffee, non-herbal teas.
- Tobacco.

DIGESTIVE AFFIRMATIONS

Say the following at least 5 times, one-half hour before meals: (Jensen, 1995)

*I eat slowly ... move slowly ... react slowly ... and my
stomach and my bowels function normally, regularly.*

I will digest my food comfortably.

My digestion is getting stronger.

My nerves are steadier and calmer.

All's well and peaceful in my life.

Indigestion. Probable cause: Gut-level fear, dread, anxiety; griping and grunting. New thought pattern: *I digest and assimilate all new experiences peacefully and joyously.*

– Louise Hay, *Heal Your Body*

Wouldst thou enjoy a long life, a healthy body, and a vigorous mind, and be acquainted also with the wonderful works of God, labor in the first place to bring thy appetite to reason.

– Benjamin Franklin

CHAPTER 5

■ ■ ■ ■ ■ ■ ■ ■ ■ ■

Intestinal Flora:
The Friendly Bacteria Story

*The much-needed "good" bacteria are of vital impor-
tance to your overall health. These bacteria are important
for the proper functioning of the metabolism, and also for
enhancing the defense mechanism of the immune system.
Lactobacillus acidophilus is a healthful bacteria that lives
in the colon. It inhibits the growth of disease-producing
bacteria and is essential for normal digestion.*

Flora are microorganisms that live, among other places, in
the bowels of humans. There are a great many of these microscopic organisms in your body and they play a crucial role in
health and disease. *The flora in the bowel is of primary importance to your state of health.* A person who is healthy and vital
invariably hosts an abundance of friendly and beneficial
microbes. A healthy intestine rich in the proper bacteria leads
to good bowel movements, vitamin processing, hormone production, and a long list of other health benefits.

If you have a healthy intestinal tract, more than 400 different
species of microorganisms are living there. They make up about
2 pounds of your body weight! Very few flora are able to survive
in the stomach because of its acidity. In fact, there may be as
few as 10 to 100 organisms in every milliliter of stomach content.
In the small intestine there may be anywhere from 100 to 1,000
organisms per milliliter. As you reach the junction between the

small and large intestine the number begins to grow. In the large intestine or colon, as many as one trillion organisms per milliliter are common.

The large bowel is in fact a mobile compost heap, constantly giving up finished compost and taking on new material for treatment. As everyone knows, a compost heap is a very special thing. Here is where the waste products of living things, both animal and vegetable, are collected for the purpose of promoting a process of decay and break-down. When the process is completed, we have the finest beginnings for a new life to get started. Out of the old and dead come the new and alive.

What is at the interface of this paradoxical phenome-non? Bacterial and micro-life forms. They are the recyclers, the transformers. They are nature's labor force, accomplishing some of the most complex chemical reactions known to man. We are constantly trying to copy or some-how utilize the processes they are capable of producing. Some of the deadliest substances in existence are produced as metabolites of these bacteria. All life upon the planet is affected by their presence. It has been determined that the colon contains not only 400 to 500 varieties of bacteria, fungi, yeast, and virus, but that the populations vary from the center of the colon to those living in the mucous lining; from those that inhabit the right side to those that inhabit the left side.

Research has found evidence to indicate that the mucous secreted by the intestine very much determines the kind of bacteria that will grow there. In addition, it has been found that it takes more than a year on the average for a new diet to produce any noticeable change in the flora.

– Excerpted from *Tissue Cleansing Through Bowel Management* by Dr. Bernard Jensen

The following is a partial list of common problems associated with inadequate bowel flora:

chronic diarrhea	*chronic bladder infections*
constipation	*intestinal gas*
breast enlargement in men	*PMS*
menstrual complaints	*dairy product allergies*
hormonal problems	*prostate troubles*
severe bruising problems	*chronic bad breath*
candida infections	*osteoporosis*
high cholesterol levels	*chronic anemia*
chronic vaginal infections	*vitamin B deficiency*

In cases of disease and decay of the body, we find large numbers of organisms that support the disease process. The body is constantly bombarded and attacked with disease-producing organisms. Lack of intestinal flora means a lack of defense against these nasties.

You can think of good intestinal maintenance as "gardening" that prepares your body with a nutritious medium in which to grow vital health. I use this analogy because, just as when we grow flowers or vegetables, we must first prepare the soil. After colonic sessions I've often told clients that we are preparing the soil. What I mean by this is that we are removing the waste material that inhibits or prevents the good, friendly bacteria from living in the bowel. If you want to grow flowers you don't just walk outside, throw the seeds up in the air, and hope they take root—chances are that few would grow. You need to prepare and nurture the soil to accept the seeds that will later result in gorgeous flowers.

It is the same with the bowel. You cannot take lactobacillus acidophilus culture, pour it onto a garbage heap, and expect the good bacteria to take root and thrive in a negative, decaying environment. I discuss intestinal flora in the colon hydro-therapy section of this book (Chapter 11), but I am also going to say it here. *Please get this!* Better yet, write it in your palm pilot or your laptop, or send yourself an e-mail: *Friendly bacteria cannot grow and thrive in a toxic environment.* If you have not done any cleansing treatment, or only minimal cleansing of your bowels, you can pretty much assume this applies to you! I swear, if one more client asks me whether having a few colonics will wash out all of the good bacteria I am going to run to the hills screaming at the top of my lungs.

ANTIBIOTIC EFFECTS ON INTESTINAL FLORA

The use of antibiotics has wreaked havoc with the intestinal ecology of humans. The widespread prescription of broad-spectrum antibiotics in our society merits our attention because of their negative effect on the beneficial organisms in our bodies.

Under the guise of traditional therapy, modern medicine can poison your body even when it is trying to heal it. Antibiotics, for example, exert a powerful negative influence on intestinal bacteria regardless of whether they are the "disease-producing" kind, or the healthy, "friendly" bacteria essential for good health. Antibiotics attack bacterial infection, but they also eradicate friendly or good bacteria needed by the body.

Bacteria lactobacillus and candida albicans (yeast organisms) are normal constituents of vaginal flora. It is not surprising, then, for a course of antibiotics to be followed by a vaginal yeast infection. Normally, the lactobacillus will keep the candida albicans under control so that it poses no threat. But, as mentioned, antibiotics throw the body out of balance, and the yeast will overgrow in the vaginal area.

We have to realize that "yeast," or candida albicans, lives in everyone's body. However, when it is stimulated by various factors, especially through use of antibiotics and birth control pills, it may establish a chronic infection known as "chronic systemic candidiasis." What happens is that the yeast is not destroyed by the use of broad-spectrum antibiotics, which kill off the friendly bacteria by the billions. Antibiotics are the worst, but they are not the only drug-induced cause of chronic candidiasis. With friendly bacteria obliterated, fungus overgrows its normal range and an individual's immune system must deal with spreading yeast. Once this candida or yeast gets into other tissues and into the bloodstream, it has the ability to overcome the immune system.

This issue is not to be taken lightly. Research suggests that candidiasis may be connected with immune disorders such as AIDS, cancer, and many other life-threatening illnesses. Anyone who has suffered with the health issue of systemic candidiasis can tell you that it is a long, hard road to reestablish the body's ecology.

WHAT YOUR DOCTOR WON'T TELL YOU

At an early age my older son, Brandon, suffered terribly from ear problems. Brandon was given antibiotics for about a year or so. I must add that as a young mother I really did not have any other information I could use to help make decisions about continual antibiotic use. Finally, I started to question the pediatrician about the recurrence of Brandon's ear problems and the constant use of antibiotics. He kept assuring me that the antibiotics were no problem at all. He convinced me to have tubes put in Brandon's ears and to have his adenoids removed. My former husband and I agreed. Here, again, is an example of a decision I would have made differently now. I started to read more about using natural therapies for healing, and in this case how to deal with infection without resorting to drugs. I learned that taking a good acidophilus after a series of anti-biotics is imperative. I asked Brandon's pediatrician about giving him acidophilus since he had been on antibiotics for over a year, but the pediatrician just laughed at me. "Oh, that is ridiculous," he said. "Your son is just fine. The antibiotics have caused no problems at all."

That was a turning point for me. I took the responsibility for getting more information, and for making decisions for my family based on natural therapies. I still wasn't a colon zealot at that time (that would come a little later), but natural supplements and herbs were sounding better all the time. I was beginning to learn. I didn't listen to that pediatrician. I did put my son Brandon on acidophilus and a full candida program to rebuild his intestinal flora and his immune system. Getting a then 8-year-old to follow a candida program, take herbs, and follow a special diet was a challenge, but he managed to get through it like a real trooper. He admitted to me later that he'd even hidden some of the herbs under the refrigerator (*that kid ...*) because he was tired of taking them. Even with his cheating, his health improved. Call it coincidence, but from about the ages of 6 and 8 my sons never saw the pediatrician: they were never really sick anymore.

Don't get me started on talking about my kids. I am a mother, after all, of two handsome sons, and we did survive the teen years (that is a book in itself) and have been through a lot together. But I could go on for days about them. What were we talking about? Oh yes, friendly bacteria.

Friendly bacteria benefit the human body in many ways. Briefly summarized, they:

1. *Acidify the colon.* The ideal pH of the colon is between 6.7 and 6.9. Acetic acid and lactic acid are some of the by-products that help create this. The acid environment inhibits the growth of harmful bacteria such as salmonella, which causes food poisoning; shigella, the main cause of diarrhea; and e. coli, which can cause intestinal disease and kidney failure. Good bacteria also produce a volatile fatty acid which, along with the other acids, makes it difficult for fungus and yeast (candida) to survive.

2. *Normalize bowel movements* by decreasing the time it takes for waste products to move through the digestive system. Good bacteria also stop diarrhea and correct constipation.

3. *Improve the immune system.* Good bacteria help stimulate the formation of antibodies that protect our bodies against infectious disease.

4. *Help produce vitamins.* Good bacteria help produce vitamin K, which is necessary for blood clotting and for the formation of new bone.

5. *Aid in production of lactase.* This enzyme is necessary to digest milk and milk products. Without lactase, milk allergies are a sure thing.

6. *Remove toxic elements.* Lactobacillus acidophilus deactivates various toxic compounds produced by other organisms or found in foods.

7. *Help reduce cholesterol.* A high-fiber diet and good bacterial flora can lower cholesterol levels, protect against colon cancer, and even improve fat digestion by providing more bile acids.

8. *Help eliminate gas problems.* Proper bacteria in the colon eliminates bowel gas and sweetens the breath. Bad breath (halitosis) is frequently caused when "bad" bacteria take over in the colon and produce foul-smelling waste. These gases can be expelled or reabsorbed into the blood and carried to the lung and exhaled. All the breath mints in the world won't correct bad breath caused by bowel problems. I knew a former neighbor who just reeked of bad breath and body odor. His wife kept asking me what supplement I could give her husband to stop his stinky breath. This woman had tried every over-the-counter remedy for halitosis known to mankind and nothing had worked. Knowing this man and his diet, I knew that his bowel was just loaded (he had what I call an "ol' poop belly"—huge and hard) from years of incorrect eating. He was not willing to

consider bowel cleansing as I'm suggesting here, so he and his bad breath (and his disappointed wife) just went on as usual. We will discuss autointoxication in Chapter 8.

Again, a proper balance of friendly bacteria is essential for optimal health and a good digestive system. An imbalance may make the body susceptible to such ailments as digestive problems, skin problems, acne, reduced immunity, arthritis, liver and gallbladder problems, failing memory, hypertension, fatigue, and migraine headaches, to name just a few.

Many people think the only reason to take lactobacillus acidophilus as a supplement is if they have some type of bowel or digestive problem. The truth is, the friendly bacteria in your bowels have some far-reaching effects you've probably never dreamed of. These hard-working organisms produce a variety of substances that can prevent cancerous tumors, inactivate viruses, produce natural antibodies and vitamins, and reduce cholesterol. New research has linked these bacteria with even more wonders.

A final note on "gardening." Keep in mind that lactobacilli acidophilus are living organisms, and as a result they are highly susceptible to dying off and losing their effectiveness. Most cultures you purchase need to be kept refrigerated or frozen to maintain their viability. There are some brands that do not have to be refrigerated (which is convenient when traveling), and they activate in the gut. They should be taken on an empty stomach 20 to 40 minutes before meals when your digestive acids and juices are not being produced in large quantities. I suggest taking these living organisms first thing in the morning on an empty stomach so they coat the intestinal tract.

Oh yes, you will need to forgo your morning cup of coffee because it will destroy all the good bacteria in your intestinal system!

CHAPTER 6

■ ■ ■ ■ ■ ■ ■ ■ ■

All About Enzymes

Food enzyme deficiencies are America's #1 nutritional problem and are responsible for more disease than all other nutritional shortages combined.

– Dr. Humbart "Smokey" Santillo

Food enzyme deficiency and its aftermath must be recognized as the most serious and profound oversight and omission in nutrition.

– Dr. Edward Howell

Life could not exist without enzymes. Enzymes are essential, but each person is born with a limited enzyme potential. Therefore, *maintaining an adequate supply of enzymes is vital to support your body's health.* Enzymes are a part of every metabolic process in the body, from the working of our glands to the proper functioning of our immune system. Enzymes not only play a role in digestion, but are also active during diseases and other metabolic processes.

When food enzymes are destroyed prior to digestion, the body must use more of its own digestive enzymes instead of relying on food enzymes to partially digest food. One of the best ways to help maintain a healthy supply of enzymes is to eat raw foods as much as possible. Not only do raw foods contain enzymes themselves, they also contain the vital co-enzymes (vitamins) that the body needs. Enzymes occurring in raw food

What Are Enzymes?

Enzymes are complex organic substances produced in plants and animals that catalyze (speed up) chemical reactions in cells and organs. There are many digestive enzymes in the body. Working with body fluids, they help to break down large chemical chains into smaller particles. The body is able to absorb these smaller food particles and utilize them. Without enzymes, body functions would be too slow to sustain life.

aid in digestion so that your body's enzymes do not have to do all the work of digestion. When you eat raw food, chewing releases the enzymes in the food to begin digestion. Then food sits in your stomach for nearly an hour before your body's digestive enzymes are secreted. It's during this time that food enzymes do their work in breaking down the complex molecules of protein, carbohydrates, fats, and fiber.

A most unfortunate characteristic of the foods we eat in our modern world is that the methods used in storing, preserving, and preparing foods kill the enzymes that are naturally found in the foods. Any kind of heat treatment of food destroys 100% of the enzymes. Baking, boiling, stewing, frying, microwaving, irradiating, etc., all completely destroy the enzymes in food. The human body and digestive system were not designed to consume cooked food. When enzymes are missing from your food, the full burden of digestion falls on your digestive system. The work of Dr. Edward Howell, a pioneer in enzyme research, has proven that a diet of cooked foods causes rapid, premature death in mice, and that the speed of premature death is directly connected to the temperature at which the food is cooked. You can reduce the enzyme destruction when cooking vegetables by using waterless cooking pans, cooking in a wok, or using a steamer.

The following is an excerpt from *Food Enzymes: The Missing Link* (second edition), written by Humbart Santillo, MH, ND:

After eating a cooked food meal, when digestive enzymes are desperately needed, the white blood cell count increases, seemingly to aid in the digestive process. Since every metabolic process is, at all times, interdependent and interrelated, this increase in the white blood cell count after the ingestion of cooked meat indicates a definite compensatory measure. The body must supply a large amount of digestive enzymes because the heating process destroyed the enzymes that were once present in the food.

Dr. Paul Kautchakoff, in his book The Influence of Food Cooking on the Blood Formula of Man, *confirms that the effects of cooked food on our systems include an increase in white blood cells, or leukocytes. (Kautchakoff, 1930)*

This increase in leukocytes is needed to transport enzymes to the digestive tract. Kautchakoff also demonstrated that after a raw food meal, there was no substantial increase in leukocytes, showing that the body has to work much harder to produce and transport enzymes for digestion after a cooked food meal.

It is important to remember that enzymes in raw food aid in the digestive process and that their action removes the stress of having to borrow them from the body's enzyme reserve, particularly from the white blood cell count that's needed to bolster your immune system.

A most important point in Kautchakoff's work is that "leukocytosis" (increased white blood cell count) is a term that describes a medical pathology. Any time the white blood cell count increases to any great extent it is likely that an acute illness or infection is present somewhere in the body. During acute diseases, enzyme levels rise. During chronic diseases, the body enzyme levels are decreased. The pancreas

and digestive tract are weakened, for example, during dia-
betes, cancer, or chronic intestinal problems.

Even though I suggest an abundance of raw foods in your daily diet to supply your digestive system with much-needed enzymes, please keep in mind that a *particular raw food provides just enough enzymes to help digest itself.* Any cooked or processed food eaten with this raw food requires supplemental enzymes to help with digestion. The body must spend great amounts of energy increasing levels of digestive enzymes to compensate for food enzymes destroyed by cooking and processing. Research suggests that eating cooked foods depletes the body's enzyme potential, and robs the body of energy needed for growth, maintenance, and repair of all of its tissues and organ systems.

Dr. Howell's studies show that the body has a genetically determined, finite enzyme potential that is gradually depleted throughout the aging process. It could be said that enzyme activity becomes weaker in old age. In his book, *Enzyme Nutrition: The Food Enzyme Concept,* Dr. Howell relates: "Dr. Meyer and his associates at Michael Reese Hospital, Chicago, found that the enzymes in the saliva of young adults was 30 times stronger than in persons over 69 years old. Dr. Eckaradt in Germany tested 1,200 urine specimens for the starch-digesting enzyme amylase. In young people it averaged 25 of his test units, and in old people, 14." (Howell, 1985)

Dr. Howell goes on to say: "There is equally prolific scientific periodical literature reporting decrease in the activity of a number of enzymes in old age." Drs. Bartos and Groh, Charles University, Prague, Czechoslovakia, enlisted as experimental subjects 10 young men and 10 men who were aged but healthy; they used a drug on all 20 men to stimulate the pancreatic juice flow. The juice was then pumped out and tested. It was found that the enzyme amylase was much weaker in the older men. Dr. Bartos, Dr. Groh, and others concluded that the enzyme deficiency of the older group was due to exhaustion of the cells of the pancreas. The real cause: "Exhaustion of the enzyme potential of the many billions of cells of the whole organism, which are depleted toward the end of life by the unnatural needs of the body's digestive juices." (Howell, 1985)

Dr. Howell's research also suggests that the rate of enzyme depletion in the body is a determining factor in longevity. Enzyme-depleted foods rob your body of its enzyme potential and may reduce your life span.

Your body gets enzymes from two main sources: internal and external. Every cell in your body is an enzyme factory. Unfortunately, the number of enzymes each cell can produce is limited. In addition, it is possible that some of us are either not born with, or lose the ability to make, certain enzymes. If we have abused our bodies with unhealthy lifestyles it is likely that deficiencies in enzymes and/or the loss of the ability to produce them will occur.

Life's demands drain your enzyme supply.

Day-to-day living puts a tremendous demand on your body's supply of enzymes. Emotional or mental strain can also adversely influence enzymatic action. Try thinking of your enzyme supply as a bank account. Skimpy deposits of enzymes (processed, dead, devitalized foods) and heavy withdrawals (chronic stress, strenuous exercise, illness) are just some of the things that can put you into eventual bankruptcy of your enzyme bank account. If you spend your enzymes rapidly, your life does not last as long as it would if you use your enzymes more frugally. The living body is under a great daily burden to produce the volume of enzymes necessary to run efficiently. Unfortunately, we are not conscious of this or we would be extremely concerned about how enzymes are dispensed, and less likely to waste them.

The digestion of enzyme-deficient food is an extremely energy-consuming task for the body. This is why we often feel tired after a big meal. Fatigue, constipation, gas, heartburn, headaches, bloating, and colon problems are just a few of the many conditions that can be caused by poor digestion and lack of enzymes.

To prevent a premature shortage of enzymes, include rich sources of enzymes in your diet whenever possible. Every bite of raw food provides your body with enzymes. Enzyme supplements taken with every meal will also add to your enzyme supply. Get in the habit of carrying supplemental enzymes with you for meals eaten outside the home. A good digestive enzyme supplement will also attempt to re-stimulate natural production of HCL (hydrochloric acid) in addition to supplementing it. One of America's biggest dietary complaints is over-acidity. Ironically, it is often caused by the lack of hydrochloric acid. When HCL is insufficient, food ferments, releasing unhealthy fermentation acids. These acids can cause ulcers and gallbladder attacks. Taking anti-acid tablets or liquids, as Americans often do, neutralizes the acids of fermentation but makes the stomach too alkaline for the normal digestion of food.

Common Digestive Supplements

papain	bromelain
lipase	bile
pepsin	pancreatin
protease	glutamic HCL
amylase	betaine HCL
lactase	

Over-the-counter digestive supplements contain other enzymes that serve various aspects of the digestive process. The papaya fruit has long had a reputation for its protein-digesting enzyme papain. Papain is found in the unripe papaya fruit and leaves. Bromelain, derived from pineapples, is another tropical fruit enzyme that helps break proteins apart into amino acids. Medical doctors have also used bromelain to clean out arteries and reduce inflammation.

Supplemental enzyme stories are not quite as glamorous as bowel cleansing treatment stories, but some bear repeating. Once, while on a lunch date (I call it my "husband interview"), I whipped out my digestive enzymes to take before we ate. My date eyed me curiously as I lined up my enzyme supplements on the table. I gave him a short explanation of why enzymes are very important with each meal. I jokingly said, "If you eat lunch with me you take enzymes with me." I scooted two of the capsules over to him, smiling. He was a good sport and took them, but he didn't seem to share my enthusiasm for food digestion. He failed the interview, by the way, but it had nothing to do with taking or not taking the enzymes!

When you add enzymes beyond what your body can produce, you can begin to rebuild your enzyme pool. Remember to keep adding generous deposits to your enzyme bank account, thus staying young and enzyme-rich for life.

CHAPTER 7

■ ■ ■ ■ ■ ■ ■ ■ ■ ■

Acid/Alkaline Balance in Body Chemistry

The term pH, which means "potential hydrogen," represents a scale for the relative acidity or alkalinity of a solution. Acidity refers to pH of 0.1 to 6.9, alkalinity is 7.1 to 14, and neutral pH is 7.0. The numbers refer to how many hydrogen atoms are present compared to an ideal or standard solution. Normally, blood is slightly alkaline, at 7.35 to 7.45. Urine pH can range from 4.8 to 7.5, although normal is closer to 7.0.

— *Alternative Medicine Definitive Guide to Cancer,*
Future Medicine Publishing, 1997

Balanced body chemistry exhibits what is called proper alkaline-acid ratio. A healthy body usually keeps large alkaline reserves to meet the demands of too many acid-producing foods. When these are depleted beyond a 4:1 ratio, health can be seriously threatened. If we eat too many acid-producing foods we become over-acid, and our immunity to disease is weakened. High acidity can affect all major body systems, especially the digestive, intestinal, circulatory, respiratory and immune systems. It is now believed that one of the basic causes of disease is acidosis, or over-acidity.

For those who have unbalanced pH and are considered "acidic," many health conditions can result. This condition forces the body to borrow minerals — including calcium, sodium, potassium and magnesium — from vital organs and bones to buffer the acid and safely remove it from the body. Over time this process can weaken these organs and bones.

ACIDOSIS MAY LEAD TO SERIOUS HEALTH CONCERNS AND AFFECT BODY SYSTEMS

The health concerns include:

◆ Cardiovascular weakness.

◆ Weight gain.

◆ Bladder and kidney concerns.

◆ Acceleration of free radical damage.

◆ Structural system weakness, including brittle bones and hip fractures.

◆ Joint discomfort and other discomfort associated with lactic acid build-up.

◆ Low energy.

A recent study conducted at the University of California, San Francisco on 9,704 post-menopausal women showed that those who have higher acidity levels (also called chronic acidosis) from a diet rich in animal foods are at a greater risk for lower bone density levels than those who have "normal" pH levels. The researchers who carried out this study hypothesized that many of the hip fractures prevalent among older women correlated to higher acidity from a diet rich in animal foods and low in vegetables. The body apparently borrows calcium from the bones in order to balance pH, and this calcium borrowing may result in a decrease in bone density

– American Journal of Clinical Nutrition
Jan. 2001, Vol. 73, No. 1, pp. 118-122

HIGH ALKALINITY IN THE BODY

Though relatively uncommon, high alkalinity in the body causes many of the same kinds of mineral problems as acidity. It often takes longer for a person who is "alkaline" to achieve balance than one who is "acidic." Alkalinity may lead to:

- ◆ Digestive system sluggishness.

- ◆ Intestinal system concerns, including poor elimination.

- ◆ Respiratory system compromise.

- ◆ Immune system weakness.

- ◆ Nervous system exhaustion.

A pH-balanced environment maintains a proper metabolism and allows the body to function optimally. In order to keep the acid-alkaline ratio in balance, Dr. Ragner Berg, the world's foremost authority on the subject, says we should eat about 80% alkaline-producing foods and 20% acid-producing foods. Alkalis help to neutralize the acids when one does become over-acidic or ill. Eating more alkaline-ash foods helps the body to maintain health and to regain a proper balanced chemistry.

ACID/ALKALINE SELF-TEST — HAVE YOU CHECKED YOUR PH TODAY?

Water is neutral with a pH of 7.0. Any pH reading below 7.0 is acid, while any pH reading above 7.0 is alkaline. The ideal range for saliva and urine is 6.0 to 6.8. Our body is naturally mildly acidic. Some people will have acidic pH readings from both urine and saliva—this is referred to as "double acid."

Urine pH

Urine testing indicates how well your body is assimilating minerals, especially calcium, magnesium, sodium, and potassium. These are called "acid buffers" because they are used by the body to control acid levels. When acid levels begin to increase, the body becomes less capable of excreting acid. It must either

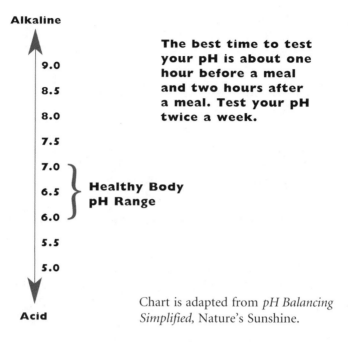

Alkaline

9.0
8.5
8.0
7.5
7.0 ⎫
6.5 ⎬ Healthy Body
6.0 ⎭ pH Range
5.5
5.0

Acid

The best time to test your pH is about one hour before a meal and two hours after a meal. Test your pH twice a week.

Chart is adapted from *pH Balancing Simplified*, Nature's Sunshine.

store the acid in body tissues or buffer it—that is, borrow minerals from organs, bones, etc., in order to neutralize the extra acid.

Acids do not stay in the blood. The body manages acids as follows:

- ◆ Excretion of acids—colon, kidneys, lungs, skin.

- ◆ Buffering of acids—calcium, magnesium, sodium, potassium.

- ◆ Storage of acids—tissue, joints, muscles, arteries.

- ◆ Minerals are used to buffer acids.

If your urinary pH *fluctuates* between 6.0 and 6.4 in the morning and 6.4 and 7.0 in the evening, your body is functioning within a normal range.

Saliva pH

The results of saliva testing indicate the activity of digestive enzymes in your body, especially the activity of the liver and the stomach. This reveals the flow of enzymes running through your body and shows their effect on all the body systems. If your saliva stays between 6.4 and 6.8 all day, your body is functioning within a normal range.

Use the lists on page 63 to adjust your diet and bring your pH balance back to normal. Alkaline-forming foods should be consumed when the body is too acidic (pH under 7.0). Acid-forming foods should be eaten when the pH is too alkaline. Low-level acid and low-level alkaline foods are almost neutral.

Although it might seem that citrus fruits would have an acid effect on the body, the citric acid they contain actually has an alkaline effect on the system, converting to carbon dioxide and water. To treat acidosis, start with small amounts of citrus fruits and gradually add larger amounts.

It is vitally important to self-test your pH levels for optimal health. pH balancing is at the foundation of your health-building program. In the privacy of your own home you can determine your pH factor quickly and easily. The Resource Guide (Chapter 24) shows you where you can order a pH testing kit.

Acid-Forming
alcohol
asparagus
beans
brussel sprouts
candy
catsup
chemical drugs
chickpeas
cocoa
coffee
cornstarch
eggs
fatty fish (sardines)
fish
flour products
legumes
lentils
meat (chicken, beef)
milk
mustard
noodles
oatmeal
olives
organ meat
pasta
pork
shellfish
smoked fish
sugar
synthetic medicines

Mildly Acid
breads
brown rice
corn
cheese
coconut (dried)
fruits (canned/glazed/dried)
grains (most)
legumes (except soybeans)
nuts (except almonds)
seeds (most)

Alkaline-Forming
almonds
apricots
avocados
beets
buckwheat
carrots
dates
fruits
grapefruit
grapes
green leafy veggies
lemons
maple syrup
melons
millet
molasses
oranges
potatoes
raisins
soybeans

Mildly Alkaline
blueberries
broccoli
cabbage
celery
green peas
lettuce
mushrooms
parsley
sesame seeds
string beans

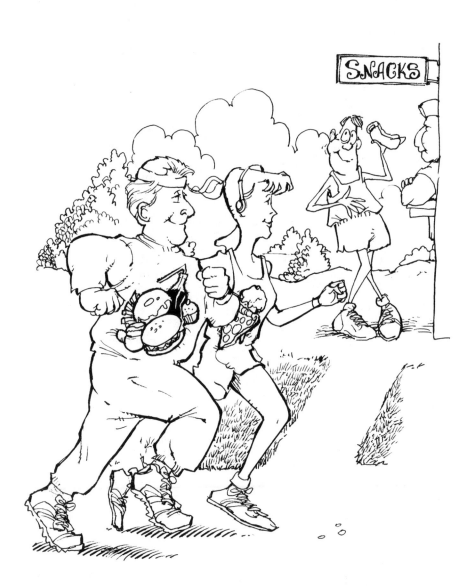

CHAPTER 8

■ ■ ■ ■ ■ ■ ■ ■ ■ ■

Autointoxication

*Pure, lasting, and abiding health is the result of
conscious discipline in cleanliness of body, mind,
and spirit. All else is compromise.*

– Bernard Jensen, DC, Ph.D., nutritionist

How much thought do you give to your colon? Probably
not very much at all. Most people take the functioning of their
digestive system for granted. As long as we *feel* reasonably well
we aren't willing to consider the tremendous impact that the
functioning of our colon can have on our overall health; a
neglected colon can be responsible for a great many of our
diseases. I am committed to sharing with you the most vital,
"kick butt" information about your health that you may ever
hear. My hope is that this information will be a big, swift "kick
in the butt" and a life-changing event.

I am very straightforward about detoxification. I have been
called many things, but *subtle* is not one of them. You will see
in no uncertain terms why I am so passionate about poop.

WHAT IS AUTOINTOXICATION?

*Autointoxication is the process whereby the body literally
poisons itself by maintaining a cesspool of decaying matter
in its colon. This inner cesspool can contain as high a
concentration of harmful bacteria as a cesspool under a
house. The toxins released by the decay process get into*

the bloodstream and travel to all parts of the body. Every cell in the body is affected, and many forms of sickness can result. Because it weakens the entire system, autointoxication can be a causative factor for nearly any disease.

– *The Colon Health Handbook*, Rockridge Publishing Co.

V. Earl Irons, a noted bowel specialist, states: "In my opinion, there is only one real disease, and that disease is *auto-intoxication*—the body poisoning itself. It is the filth in our system that kills us. So I am convinced that unless you clean out your bowel you will never reach vibrant health." Many of the health problems we "live with" are problems we can control by getting rid of stagnating and fermenting foods that should have been removed as waste from our body but instead are collecting inside. The possibility of attaining any degree of vibrant health is lost if such fermentation occurs, accumulates, and is retained by the body. If we are to attain any degree of health, we must not allow the intestines to remain loaded with waste material.

The average person carries around 10 to 15 pounds of fecal matter in their intestines. Think about that for a minute: 10 to 15 pounds of disgusting crud rotting in your guts. It has been stated that actor John Wayne's colon weighed an incredible 60 pounds at his death. Can you imagine *your* colon weighing 60 pounds? We have an example of an autopsy revealing another colon weighing in at an incredible 40 pounds. Are you starting to get the picture here?

The very best of diets can be no better than the very worst, if the sewage system of the colon is clogged with a collection of waste and corruption.

– Norman Walker, D.Sc., Ph.D.

MEDICAL OPINION

◆ "No harm can result if 1 to 10 days pass without a normal bowel movement."

◆ "The range of normal varies from 3 movements a day to one every 2 weeks."

◆ "You may not have a bowel movement for 7 days or 10 days or even 20 days. The material accumulated in your colon is not dangerous to your health. Anticipate and accept twinges and the distended belly that will result. It is worth the wait."

ALTERNATIVE OPINION

Any doctor or health professional who is interested in a natural approach to better health will always place great emphasis on elimination, transit time, autointoxication, and cleansing. Because a difference in opinion exists, I'll let you decide. Even one movement per day means that 3 meals' worth of waste is still in the colon at all times. How would you feel if 2 weeks' worth of meals were backed up in your system? That's 42 meals without movement! You decide which is better: eliminating once or twice daily, or once every 2 weeks.

Autointoxication, or toxemia, is a form of self-poisoning, and one of the most prevalent conditions that acts as a barrier to good health. As such it becomes the seat of many diseases, according to the clinical studies of many eminent doctors. These physicians include John H. Tilden, MD; Rasmus Alsaker, MD; Frank McCoy, DC; M.O. Gartens, DC; Bernard Jensen, Ph.D., DC; Norman Walker; and many others whose widely known writings are up-to-date and still available.

In his popular work, *Toxemia Explained*, Dr. Tilden says:

> *Without toxemia there can be no disease. All diseases are the same fundamentally. The cause travels back to toxemia, caused by enervation (lack of nerve energy), which*

checks elimination and induces a toxic state. Every chronic disease starts with toxemia and a toxic crisis. When the nervous system is normal—when there is nerve energy— man is normal and immune to disease. Disease begins to manifest only when environments and personal habits use up energy faster that it is renewed.

The late Dr. Bernard Jensen, DC, a natural healer of international renown, summarizes the results of his experience:

In the 50 years I've spent helping people to overcome disability and disease, it has become crystal clear that poor bowel management lives at the root of most people's health problems. In treating over 500,000 patients, it is the bowel that invariably has to be cared for before effective healing can take place. Trying to take care of any symptom in the body without good elimination is futile.

DR. CARRELL'S EXPERIMENT

In 1911, Dr. Alexis Carrell of the Rockefeller Institute successfully grew living chicken tissue cells on microscope slides for the first time. Receiving the Nobel Prize for this and other research, Dr. Carrell was able to keep tissue cells alive through daily nutritious feedings. By washing away the tissue evacuation, the cells grew and thrived. However, he found that if the evacuations were left for 3 days, the cells died. *Interesting.* In spite of daily feedings, moderate saturation of the tissue cells by their digestive evacuations resulted in lowered vitality. Prolonged unsanitary conditions brought death to the cells.

Just as in Dr. Carrell's experiment with living chicken tissue cells, the tissue cells of our bodies will possess lowered vitality and resisting power if supplied with impure blood. Disease and degeneration result in tissue cells that are invaded and affected by the insidious behavior of microorganisms and their poisonous toxins. Even though the cells and tissues comprising our anatomy are live organisms with an amazing degree of resilience, they must still be nourished. To replenish and re-invigorate these cells and tissues, nourishment must necessarily be composed of live elements (i.e., foods with life-giving properties).

INTERNAL TOXEMIA

The body has a great deal of additional waste to dispose of through the colon in the form of used-up cells and tissues. These cells and tissues are dead proteins — highly toxic if allowed to ferment and putrefy in the intestinal system. The body constantly regenerates and grows new tissues and cells; it also produces toxins through normal, everyday functions that, in turn, continually add to waste within our body. Our body has to metabolize this waste. The concern here is due to the excess intake or production of toxins in the body, and the reduction in the efficiency of the elimination process. Toxicity occurs when we ingest more than we can utilize and excrete through the body's designed eliminative channels (bowels, kidneys, lungs, skin, lymphatic system). The end result can be serious illness.

ALIMENTARY TOXEMIA

The subject of alimentary toxemia was discussed in London, before the Royal Society of Medicine, by 57 of the leading physicians of Great Britain. Among the speakers were eminent surgeons, physicians, and specialists in the various branches of medicine. Several speakers noted the various poisons (36) of alimentary intestinal toxemia and their effects on the body. It was stated that "of these 36 poisons several are highly active, producing most profound effects, and in very small quantities. In cases of alimentary toxemia some of these poisons are continually bathing the delicate body cells and setting up changes which finally result in grave disease."

Death Begins in the Colon

The colon is a sewage system, but by neglect and abuse it becomes a cesspool. When it is clean and normal we are well and happy. Let it stagnate and it will distill the poisons of decay, fermentation, and putrefaction into the blood, poisoning the brain and nervous system so that we become mentally depressed and irritable; it will poison the heart so that we are weak and listless; poison the lungs so that the breath is foul; poison the digestive organs so we are distressed and bloated; and poison the blood so the skin is sallow and unhealthy. In short, every organ of the body is poisoned, and we age prematurely; look and feel old; the joints are stiff and painful; neuritis, dull eyes, and a sluggish brain overtake us; and the pleasure of living is gone.

— Jensen, 1974

If you think autointoxication does not have any correlation with illness and disease, think again. Colds and flu are the body's way of removing toxins through their symptoms of diarrhea, vomiting, fevers, running noses, etc. Your body is trying to tell you something. Your body is toxic and is trying to get well. *Listen to it!* Let your body perform its own healing miracles. It's trying to cleanse itself. Get out of your own way.

Hopefully, you have picked up this book before a life-threatening health challenge drives you to make changes. You might be considering detoxification as a prevention/maintenance effort. If you think you are *above* getting a colonic treatment, or giving yourself an enema, or whatever it takes to get well, *get over yourself!* It's all part of helping your body to heal itself. The body's way of healing itself (retracing disease) will be discussed at greater length in Chapter 19.

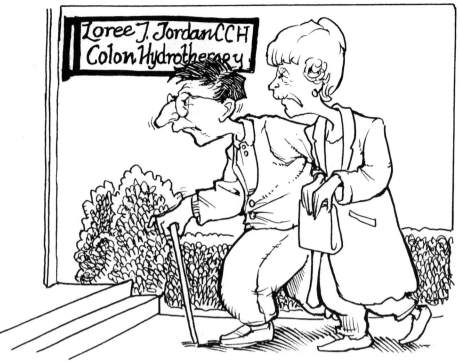

Before the Colonic

Is This You?

Some common symptoms of toxicity overload in the body:

constipation	*headaches*
depression	*acne*
fatigue	*skin conditions (eczema, psoriasis, etc.)*
frequent colds	*sinus congestion*
halitosis (bad breath)	*joint stiffness/aches and pains*
indigestion	*menstrual problems*
obesity	*allergies*

All the "itis's" — colitis, diverticulitis, bronchitis, pancreatitis, sinusitis, etc.

A LESSON FROM LUCY

I always remember Lucille Ball fondly for one episode from *I Love Lucy*. The episode showed her at work in a factory. Her job was to package candies going by on a conveyer belt. The point of using this metaphor (besides that this was a hilarious skit by a brilliant actress) is that she could not keep up with the candies coming down the belt. The candies were piling up and falling off the belt onto the floor. She got so overwhelmed that she tried to keep up by shoving them into her mouth. She was trying everything she could, in vain, to keep up with the conveyer belt and to manage the backup of candies.

Our bodies are like that factory. The processing mechanism (Lucy and her boxes) becomes overwhelmed by the flow of devitalized foods (the candies). Like Lucy, our body can only keep up the race for so long before things start to break down. Our bodies, given their various inherent strengths and weaknesses, manage quite well with the substances we put into them, and with the activities of work and play that make up our lives. But why push it? Give Lucy a break.

NUTRITIONAL ABUSE

The majority of people have eaten incorrectly since childhood, with bad habits continuing through adulthood. Usually it is not until a health issue arises—either minor (such as wanting to trim down and lose weight) or life-threatening—that we choose to really examine our eating habits and possible nutritional abuse.

The food that we ingest is basically fuel to operate, maintain, and repair our body. The body was designed to be able to survive and thrive on a long list of what the earth provides for us, but this list does not include *everything* represented as food these days. Most of us do not live off the land as our ancestors did. Great-great-great-grandpa John would not have snacked on Twinkies and Doritos while riding in an air-conditioned

Devitalized food is often "easy" and convenient, but it leads to a devitalized life and a low level of health. The body was not designed to cope with chemical additives, preservatives, artificial colors, flavoring, and so forth, but functions most effectively on fresh fruits, vegetables, grains, nuts, seeds, and other foods, prepared in such a manner that their nutrient value is not impaired or destroyed. I say "live foods, live body ... dead foods, dead body!" The whiter the bread ... the quicker you're dead!

tractor cab, or come out of the barn with a triple mocha latté made with cream from the farm cow. Our bodies are not designed for the diets we have grown accustomed to. That is why I believe we are in disease and toxicity crises, and detoxification now is more critical than ever.

FIBER FOODS

There are numerous food substances whose ultimate function is to cleanse and remove used-up cells and tissues and take this waste matter to the colon for evacuation from the body. One of these foods is fiber. Fiber is extremely important to the digestive system. Fiber, however, must be composed of roughage, that which is found in raw foods. When these fibers pass through the intestines they become, figuratively speaking, highly magnetized, and in this condition are very helpful in the functions involved in the various parts of the intestines. This fiber acts like an intestinal broom.

In contrast, when "demagnetized" or dead, devitalized foods pass through the body's digestive system, the cumulative effect can be a coating like a sticky, gluey paste on the inner walls of the colon. Over time this coating may gradually increase its thickness until there is only a small hole through the center. In severe cases this opening can shrink to the diameter of a pencil, through which the feces is supposed to pass. One autopsied colon measured 9 inches wide (normal width is 2½ inches), and this woman had professed to be eliminating 5 times a day!

DENIAL ... IS NOT A RIVER IN EGYPT

"No way is that stuff inside of me," you exclaim! If you do not believe this black, thick, rubberlike lining can exist in your body, go back and reread my personal experience in the first chapter of this book. If anyone doubted the possibility of such a foul surprise lurking in their system, *it was me!*

Talk about a life-changing event. The experience of dropping about 10 pounds of the most revolting black material I have ever seen in my own bathroom has altered my perspective. *There is no substitute for experience!* But don't just take my word for it. Pick up a copy of *Tissue Cleansing Through Bowel Management* by Dr. Bernard Jensen and study those disgusting pictures of putrid bowel material. It will give you nightmares. While a picture may be worth a thousand words, you will probably be left speechless, your mouth gaping open, to gasp or scream. Please read Chapter 16, "Real People, Real Stories," for testimonials from people just like you who found out (much to their amazed horror) that they were "full of it" and didn't even know it.

NATURE'S PROTECTIVE MECHANISM

So you are probably asking yourself: What exactly is this black, putrid, hardened mucous? Where does it come from? How does it form on the insides of the folds and crevices of colon wall? Well, according to V. Earl Irons, it results from the violation—from 1 to 3 times every day since you were two years old—of two major natural laws.

The first natural law violation is eating the wrong combination of foods. Please refer to Chapter 3 and the chart on proper food combining. Food combining is essential to avoid putrefaction of food during the digestive process. The second natural law violation is the constant daily consumption of tremendous amounts of dead, devitalized foods. Any food that is not a raw fruit or vegetable (high water-content food) is considered to be a dead/devitalized food. According to Irons:

The wrong application of both of these laws has caused the body's natural protective mechanism to secrete mucous into the colon to protect the body from absorbing the many poisons which those counterfeit foods create. But we have simply overworked nature's protective mechanism to the point that the mechanism, instead of protecting us from poisons, now poisons us.

You see, nature's protective mechanism was not designed for the enormous and continuous use to which it has been subjected. It was designed to protect us from the occasional ingestion of poisonous food that ordinarily might happen only once or twice a month, or less. When food that is not wholesome or is harmful to the body reaches the stomach, word is immediately sent from the stomach to the mucous manufacturer, warning: "Get busy, the enemy is on the way." The way in which the message is sent is immaterial. We do know that mucus production starts immediately, and the colon is lined with it. When the poisoned or harmful food from the stomach finally enters the colon 12 to 18 hours later, the latter is well prepared with a layer of mucous lining, so the body does not absorb any of the poisons. Were that to happen once or even several times a month, this mucous, having served its purpose, would disintegrate and slowly be discharged from the colon with no harm done.

But it is now apparent that nature never intended this protective mechanism to see continuous use, as it does today. This protective mechanism was never designed to continue secreting mucous, one layer on top of another layer for years, with no time out or chance for its elimination. The result is that layer on top of layer is secreted until its accumulation thickens to ⅛- to ¼-inch thick. Sometimes this layer gets ⅜- to ½-inch thick, becoming as hard and black as the piece of old, discarded rubber you see on a highway from a blown truck tire.

It is horrible to realize how we abuse nature's protective mechanism, damaging it to the point where it becomes toxic itself, and is a continuous disease-producer. To be sure, the waste product of normal metabolism is toxic, and the only reason we are not poisoned by it is because it is removed from the body as fast as it is produced. This is not the case with this hardened mucous. It is not removed but lies imbedded in the vast folds of the colon, continuously emitting toxins—creating toxemia and autointoxication— the primary cause of most all disease.

I need to emphasize here that, even though we have been talking primarily about the large intestine (the colon), the small intestine can also build up a lining or "plaque" that must also be cleansed. This plaque in the small intestine can impair nutrient absorption. The little fingers of the villi in the small intestine cannot extract the nutrients they need if this plaque or sheath is present.

All of my research over the years has shown that there is documented proof that toxic material builds up in the colon. However, many will state that the "black sludge" that is removed from the body may possibly be coming from the small intestine as well.

CONSTIPATION DEFINED

Many clients have expended a lot of energy trying to convince me that they are not constipated, even though they may

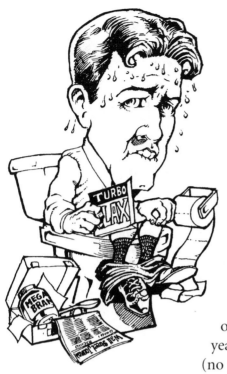

have only one bowel movement per day. Many years ago I, too, was under that same impression with regard to my, uh, movements. But again, experience has led me to believe otherwise. In my own experience I was uninformed about how a clean bowel should function, and was unaware that I was actually constipated.

Let's do the math here. If you eat an average of 3 meals a day and poop only once a day, in the course of a year you are 730 meals behind (no pun intended). Just like Lucy and all the candies backing up on the conveyer belt, you now have 730 meals' worth of foods backing up ... guess where? You got it ... in your intestines. Think of the poor souls who poop only every few days or go weeks without a bowel movement. Believe me, these people exist. You may even be one of them!

If you eat 3 meals a day you should be pooping 3 times a day. If your digestive system is working properly you should have a bowel movement soon after eating a meal. Anything less than that is considered constipated. So, really, what is the

Proper intestinal management is probably one of the most important things a person can learn in a health-building lifestyle, since some of the most important functions relating to our health take place in the colon.

77

definition of constipation? The term *constipation* is derived from the Latin word *constipatus,* which means "to press or crowd together, to pack, to cram." Consequently, to be constipated means that the packed accumulation of feces in the bowel makes evacuation difficult. However, a state of constipation can also exist when movements of the bowel *seem* normal in spite of an accumulation of feces somewhere in the large intestine.

Diarrhea is also a form a constipation. It is the body's way of trying to get rid of impacted matter further up in the colon.

PRIMARY CAUSES OF CONSTIPATION

Some of the primary causes of constipation are:

◆ *Unconscious nutrition.* Processed, devitalized foods low in natural fiber or bulk are not suitable substances to promote health and well-being.

◆ *Ignoring the call to eliminate.* Feces or urine contribute greatly to cellular congestion, autointoxication, and eliminative organ distress. Intestinal constipation causes cellular constipation. It also increases the workload of the excretory organs (the kidney, skin, liver, lungs, and lymph). The functioning of these organs becomes stressed and overworked. The cellular metabolism becomes sluggish, repair and growth are delayed, and the ability to eliminate waste materials is lowered. Instead of being alive and active, the cells become dead and inactive. This process results in a decline in functional ability of tissues and organs.

◆ *Lack of physical exercise/sedentary lifestyle.* Lack of exercise results in weak and flaccid muscles incapable of holding up under the demands of poor, inadequate diets and the extra eliminative burden placed on the body. Many people have what is called an "atonic" bowel, where the bowel is not performing adequate peristalsis (muscular contractions that move food along the tube of the colon to the rectum). Dr. Bernard

Jensen refers to this as a "Twinkie" bowel. To treat it the bowel has to become re-toned and shaped up after years of abuse and inactive lifestyle.

◆ *Emotional/mental stress and strain.* Stress produces unfavorable conditions in the digestive and eliminative organs, causing them to become tense and underactive. A relaxing environment is essential for adequate digestion.

◆ *Consumption of poisons.* Poisons (such as tobacco, coffee, alcohol, chocolate, and sugar) have unfavorable effects upon digestion and elimination by upsetting gastric secretions and nerve responses. Some medications have a very upsetting effect upon these life-giving functions. Medications may cause many afflictions in the bowel. Medications also place severe stress on the filtering process of the liver. Laxatives should be considered poisons and can be very irritating to the bowel.

◆ *Inadequate water consumption.* Most people do not drink enough water and are chronically dehydrated. This causes body tissues and fluids to become thicker. The mucus lining in the colon changes in consistency, failing to provide a slick lubrication for the movement of the feces.

◆ *Poor living habits.* Not following a good health program contributes a great deal to poor bowel function by denying the body regularity and consistency. It never knows what's coming next and can't depend upon a regular routine. It is always on the defensive. The result of this is a depletion of vital nerve force, and an undermining of the body's ability to set periods of rest and activity.

According to V. Earl Irons, a nationally known colon specialist, you are constipated when less than 100% of the food you ate in the last 24 to 48 hours comes out when you go to the bathroom. If you are completely healthy and have a completely healthy colon, 100% of the food you eat will come out within 24 to 48 hours of eating. But the big question to ask, he says, is: "Does all the food which is supposed to come out, come out?" In most people, all the food they eat *does not* come out within 24 to 48 hours after a meal. In many cases, food stays in a person for months and even years.

This food will rot, decay, and get buried in the crevices and folds of the colon; it can stay in the body for 10 years or more. Healthview Newsletter asked V. Earl Irons if food could actually stay in the body for that length of time.

> *You are darn right it can. Sometimes even longer. Some people still have a part of the turkey dinner in them which they ate at Grandma's 10 years ago. Pieces of the white meat, potatoes, and stuffing are still "stuffed" in them. It might sound funny, but it is not a laughing matter.* (Healthview, 1983)

Louise Hay identifies the possible emotional component of constipation as follows: (Louise Hay, *Heal Your Body*)

> *Constipation.* Probable cause: Refusing to release old ideas, stuck in the past. Sometimes stinginess. New thought pattern: *As I release the past, the new and fresh and vital enter. I allow life to flow through me.*

> *Bowel problems.* Probable cause: Resent the release of waste. New thought pattern: *I freely and easily release the old, and joyously welcome the new.*

DIFFERENCES OF OPINION

I love V. Earl Irons's answer when asked, "Does the medical profession agree with your views that any health problems can be caused by a toxic colon?"

> *I doubt it. The medical profession knows very little about the colon. Most doctors are ignorant on the subject—totally ignorant. In my opinion, most medical doctors should have*

their licenses taken away until they start to treat the real cause of most people's problems: a diseased colon.

He goes on to say that most of the drugs, medicines, and operations given today have never made any person's colon one bit healthier. If anything, they have only made the situation worse:

> *You know, it is interesting that before the turn of the century, most medical doctors did understand something about the importance of a clean colon. Why today, if you just mention the word "colon" to your doctor, he will most likely just laugh at you. You can be dead and long buried, and even then your doctor would never admit that your clogged colon had anything at all to do with your ill health. (Healthview, 1983)*

Refer to Chapter 12, "What Other Health Professionals Are Saying," to learn how V. Earl Irons's son, Robert Irons, has carried on his father's legacy.

MEDICAL OBJECTIONS TO COLON CLEANSING

Medical objection: The body cleanses itself naturally. There is no need for any special cleansing program. Cleansing the colon is dangerous and completely unnecessary.

My response: Considering the inadequate, devitalized foods most people eat today, there is no way the colon can cleanse itself "naturally." If we ate an adequate diet, consisting of plenty of natural, raw foods, yes, the body would be able to cleanse itself. The real danger here is trying to live a long healthy life with 10 to 15 pounds of fecal matter backed up in the colon.

If the colon cleanses itself naturally, then why is more than $400 million a year spent on laxatives in the U.S.? Why do more than 70 million Americans suffer from bowel problems? Why do 100,000 people undergo colostomies each year in the U.S.?

There is but one cause of disease—poison or toxemia, most of which is created in the body by faulty living habits and faulty elimination.

– Major General Sir Arbuthnot Lane, MD

If the colon cleanses itself naturally, then why do people rid themselves of pounds of putrid fecal matter and impacted mucus upon completing a bowel cleansing program?

Medical objection: Wastes accumulating in the colon are not toxic.

My response: The intestinal system is a porous organ (such as the colon) and in fact releases toxins into the entire body via the bloodstream and the lymphatic system.

If you ask the average physician about autointoxication, trust me, s/he will most likely downplay your concerns. The average doctor in general does not have any concept of how to detoxify the body, and most certainly does not relate it to disease control. Of course, there are also many doctors who do support detoxification. My intent is not to criticize the medical profession. It provides a great service, but many practitioners are just not trained to new concepts in the field of nutrition and disease prevention through detoxification.

I think V. Earl Irons could not have said it better: "The medical profession labels any form of therapy as quackery if they themselves are not able to administer or control it." I would like to take that comment one step further and say that, if there is no financial gain on their part, they are really going to shout "quackery."

I believe in detoxification like I believe in air, and I am truly passionate about poop. I have absolutely no doubt in my mind that autointoxication is at the root of much of our ill health and disease.

You wouldn't even consider going weeks without a shower or brushing your teeth (at least I hope you wouldn't). So why would you go for years without cleansing your internal system? There are viable solutions to the autointoxication dilemma. Our goal here should be to detoxify the whole body system in order to rebuild and regenerate new cells and tissue. We want to grow younger, with a new body, and not stay in a diseased, toxic body. Don't we? The promise of this book is to show you how.

CHAPTER 9

■ ■ ■ ■ ■ ■ ■ ■ ■

Cancer

We are not winning the war against cancer. We are losing the war. The number of Americans getting cancer each year has escalated over recent decades, while our ability to treat and cure most common cancers has remained virtually unchanged.

– Samuel S. Epstein, MD

BUYER BEWARE: YOUR RIGHT TO KNOW

I now want to focus on how diet and ingested toxins contribute to cancer. I do not want to minimize or discount other contributors to carcinogenic statistics (such as environmental, airborne, work-related toxins, etc.). But for the purpose of this book I have streamlined our focus to ingested foods, beverages, and chemical toxins.

As consumers we have a right to know what ingredients are in the food products we use and ingest daily. We try to make educated and intelligent choices based on food labeling. We want to be accurately informed about any chemicals which could pose a chronic health risk to our families and ourselves, before we make a purchasing decision.

Until now, however, most of us have been shopping in the dark. We have been receiving little guidance from food producers and product manufacturers, whose advertising and labeling are not objective and are often misleading. It takes a lot of time and energy to become a label sleuth and to really examine which chemicals and additives we have in our foods.

Buyer beware: your life depends on it. If you are an avid label reader you may already know how minimal regulation has led to grossly inadequate labeling.

When was the last time your supermarket warned you which fish or other food product or packaging contained chemicals that cause cancer or birth defects? Food and beverages may be contaminated with a variety of chemicals that have been, intentionally or unintentionally, added during their production, handling, storage, and processing. Fruits, vegetables, nuts, seeds, and grains are contaminated primarily with pesticides, and sometimes mold. Dairy, meat, seafood, and processed foods are also contaminated with industrial chemicals, additives, hormones, growth stimulants, antibiotics, and other animal drugs, as well as occasionally mold and bacteria. Many, if not all, of these chemicals have carcinogenic, neurotoxic, reproductive, or immunotoxic effects. These chemicals are a threat to your health, and to your children's health.

Without exception one of the favorite foods of American children is hot dogs. I say, "Hold the hot dogs!" Samuel Epstein, MD, seems to share my opinion when he states that children who eat hot dogs containing nitrate preservatives (which are precursors of carcinogenic nitrosamines) about a dozen times a month have up to fourfold excess risk of brain cancer and a sevenfold excess risk of leukemia.

There was a lot of go-around and wrangling with my sons over this subject but I always held my ground. At a theme park my former husband bought the boys hot dogs while I was off looking at something else. I am sure he felt between a rock and a hard place, with two kids whining for hot dogs and a wife who was very displeased with his decision.

Pesticides in the Diets of Infants and Children, issued by the National Academy of Sciences, and *Pesticides in Children's Food,* prepared by the Environmental Working Group, a Washington-

> *An overemphasis on the diagnosis and treatment of
> cancer and relative neglect of its prevention, coupled
> with ineffective regulation of carcinogens in air, water,
> food, consumer products, and the workplace, have
> contributed to escalating cancer rates and an annual
> death toll of over 500,000. The National Cancer
> Institute and the American Cancer Society, which
> should be the chief advocates of cancer prevention,
> instead mislead the public and policy-makers into
> believing that we are winning the war against cancer,
> and trivialize the role of avoidable exposures to
> industrial carcinogens.*
>
> – *The Politics of Cancer Revisited*, Epstein, 1998

based nonprofit research organization, both concluded that
infants and children are at high risk for future cancers because
of their exposure to carcinogenic pesticides.

Adults are also at risk, from both their childhood and current exposures to chemical contaminants. A 1993 study found
that women with the highest levels of DDT had 4 times the
risk of breast cancer than women with the lowest exposure.
This study is only one of many since the 1970s — all largely
unpublicized — to associate DDT and other related pesticides
and industrial chemicals with breast cancer risk. In fact, there
is growing evidence that the nation's present breast cancer epidemic is related to exposure to a wide range of environmental
contaminants, including DDT, other carcinogenic pesticides,
and estrogenic stimulants.

Consumers (like you and me) who have questioned the
presence of carcinogen residues in the food supply have been
told that the amounts are trivial and there is no cause for
concern. When cancer statistics are going up, not down, and

when 1 in 3 Americans is now stricken with cancer (in 1950 it was 1 in 4), reducing our exposure to carcinogenic substances deserves immediate attention.

Change is coming, and many citizens have decided to boycott foods and beverages contaminated with carcinogens that pose health risks. We have only scratched the surface. It is going to take a lot more consumer outrage and action. The FDA has to be pushed to require labeling foods for carcinogenic pesticides and other contaminants. Meanwhile it is up to you, and you alone, to take responsibility to educate and arm yourself with knowledge and minimize your exposure.

CARCINOGENS IN FOODS AND BEVERAGES

The following is a list of some known carcinogens in our foods and beverages. (Epstein, 1998)

Artificial colors. Citrus red #2, used to dye the skins of Florida oranges, is carcinogenic.

Fruits. Most fruits are contaminated with a wide range of carcinogenic pesticides. Buy organically grown produce whenever possible!

Unwitting exposure of the entire U.S. population to avoidable carcinogens continues to play an important causal role in escalating cancer rates. However, the cancer establishment has remained silent about these exposures, which are well documented in the scientific literature, and has failed to testify before Congress or advise the regulatory agencies concerned. The American Cancer Society has actually gone still further, in trivializing these risks and opposing their regulation.

– The Safe Shoppers Bible

Vegetables. Like fruits, most vegetables are also contaminated with a wide range of carcinogenic pesticides. Buy organic vegetables whenever possible.

Meat and poultry. Meat and poultry contain a wide range of carcinogens, including pesticides, animal drugs, hormones (given to 95% or more of the cattle raised for slaughter in the U.S.), and radiation. Many of these carcinogens remain in the tissues of the animal and end up on your plate! It is wise to know your meat source. Buy only hormone-free and free-range meats at your local health food store.

Waxes. Waxes contain fungicides such as benomyl and sodium orthophenyl phenate; both are carcinogenic. Fruits and vegetables may be waxed for better visual presentation.

Dairy products. Dairy products contain many carcinogenic pesticides including BHC, chlordane, DDT, dieldrin, heptachlor, HCB, and indane, which accumulate in the most fatty dairy products (e.g., butter, ice cream, whole milk, high-fat cheeses). The Health Protection Branch of Canada has reported dioxin levels in the part-per-trillion range in several samples of milk and cream packaged in bleached milk cartons manufactured in the United States. Dioxin, a byproduct of the process used to bleach paper, had migrated from the carton to the milk. Very likely U.S. milk products are similarly contaminated with dioxin. Dioxin's carcinogenicity is up to 500,000 times more potent than that of DDT.

Additives. Some additives such as coal tar, food colors, potassium bromate, and BHA are carcinogenic, or have shown suggestive evidence of carcinogenicity.

Preserved foods. Preserved foods, especially in processed food containing cured meats, such as pepperoni pizza, sausages, and luncheon meats, can be carcinogenic. The presence of nitrate preservatives deserves caution. Nitrates interact with other secondary tertiary amines — in the food (especially following cooking) and in the stomach—to form carcinogenic nitrosa-mines. There *are* safer alternatives available. Avoid all processed and preserved foods.

Processed foods. Processed foods contain concentrations of carcinogenic pesticides. Brands using organic ingredients are preferable.

Vegetable oils. Although most oils tend to be free from carcinogenic pesticide residues, soybean oil is contaminated with residues of dieldrin. Safflower oil is contaminated with lindane, which is carcinogenic. Oils that are improperly stored can become oxidized, leading to formation of oxygen-free radicals that are associated with carcinogenic processes.

Artificial sweeteners. Aspartame is used in Equal and Nutra-Sweet, as well as many brands of low-calorie diet foods, desserts, and soft drinks. There are many studies pending to determine aspartame's possible association with brain tumors.

Drinking water. A major cancer risk, arsenic contaminates the drinking water of millions of Americans. Other water contaminants found to be carcinogenic are fluoride, industrial pollutants, lead, pesticides, and radiation. Some experts believe that the plastic used to store water and soft drinks contains dimethylterephthalate and is carcinogenic.

COLON CANCER

Colorectal cancer strikes 130,000 men and women each year in the U.S.

– American Cancer Society

What do Charles Schultz (creator of Peanuts), Katie Couric, actress Audrey Hepburn, and baseball player Darryl Strawberry have in common? They have all been touched by colon cancer. Katie Couric is on a national crusade to make the public aware of preventative colon screening tests for colon cancer after losing her husband Jay (age 42) to colon cancer in 1998.

In Western countries the colon and rectum account for more new cases of cancer every year than any other anatomical site except for the lung. In the USA approximately 60,000 people will die of this disease in 1986. About 70% of these cancers occur in the rectum and sigmoid colon. Cancer of the colon and rectum is the second most frequent cause of death among visceral malignancies that affect both sexes. The incidence increases with age, beginning to rise at age 40 and reaching a peak at 60 to 75 years. Carcinoma (cancer) of the colon is more common in females, and carcinoma (cancer) of the rectum is more common in males. Synchronous colonic cancers (more than one cancer) are found in 5% of the patients. There is a low genetic predisposition to cancer of the large bowel, but "cancer families" and "colon cancer families" are described in which colorectal cancer occurs across several generations, usually present before age 40, and occurs more commonly in the right colon. Other predisposing factors include chronic ulcerative colitis, graulomatous colitis, and familial polyposis; in these disorders, the risk of cancer is related to the age of onset and duration of the underlying disease. Populations with a high incidence of colorectal cancer consume diets containing less fiber and more animal protein, fat, and refined carbohydrates than populations with a low incidence of the disease.

Signs and symptoms of colon cancer include rectal bleeding, change in bowel habits, abdominal cramping or pain, blood in the stool, unexplained anemia, and weight loss. There is an increased risk of colon cancer when colon polyps, or ulcerative bowel disease exist. Methods for early detection of polyps and tumors include rectal exam, sigmoidoscopy, and stool testing for microscopic blood. Definitive diagnosis is made by x-ray, endoscopy of the colon, and biopsy.

– Merck Manual (15th edition), 1987

Research indicates that 2 out of every 3 cases of colorectal cancer are detectable by colonoscopy and sigmoidoscopy. If detected early, dietary treatment, along with the other alternative therapies such as those recommended in *The Definitive Guide to Cancer,* may constitute the most appropriate line of attack. Remember, I am holistically minded. If you are looking for suggestions on chemotherapy and radiation for cancer I can tell you, you have the wrong book in your hands. I wish you the best on your journey, but I am on a different path.

The #1 risk factor for colorectal cancer is the consumption of red meat (but not fish or white meat), Refined sugar-containing foods, or white flour products. A diet low in fruits and vegetables also increases risk. According to *The Definitive Guide to Cancer,* dietary antioxidants (notably vitamin E), calcium, vitamin D, and the B-vitamin folic acid (folate) may also reduce risk or even aid in reversing this cancer in its early stages.

Colorectal cancer (cancers of either the colon or rectum) is the second most common cancer in the U.S. and surely one of the deadliest. In fact, about 1 out of every 5 cancer deaths (20% in the U.S.) is attributed to colorectal cancer and almost half of all colorectal patients will die, according to conventional medical statistics.

– The Alternative Definitive Guide to Cancer, 1997

CANCER AND AUTOINTOXICATION

Women who have 2 or fewer bowel movements per week have 4 times the risk of breast disease as women who have 1 or more bowel movements per day.

– Saturday Evening Post

So what does cancer have to do with autointoxication? In my opinion, everything. Statistics show that cancer (excluding about 5% from genetic factors) can be a direct result of the level of autointoxication in a person's body. The bowel history and dietary factors are of primary importance in determining cancer risk factors. One of the greatest risks a human being can take is to allow fecal end products to remain in contact with the lining of the colon for 3 to 4 days at a time. Again, to quote J.J. Tilden, MD, in *Toxemia Explained:* "Without toxemia there can be no disease."

It would be ignorant and irreverent to claim that colonic cleansing alone could cure cancer. But consider the regimens employed in most of the alternative cancer therapy clinics, and notice that practically all emphasize the role of a toxic colon in the genesis of cancer. Some employ colon cleansing methods many times a day, with the addition of rectal implants.

CANCER PATIENTS IMPROVE FROM RECEIVING COLON TREATMENT

"I have found over the years that cancer patients who are not doing well usually are toxic and not being cleansed. They certainly are in need of colon hydrotherapy," advises oncologist and homeopath Douglas Brodie, MD, of Reno, Nevada. Dr. Brodie has developed CAM (complementary alternative modalities) methods for treating cancer and other degenerative diseases aimed at strengthening the immune system. He emphasizes natural and humane approaches to these conditions with colon hydrotherapy being among them.

"I do recommend that most of my cancer patients take colon hydrotherapy or 'colonic irrigations' because they often improve by having such treatment. Liver cancer in particular shows benefit from colon hydrotherapy, but any internal tumors show effectual change too," Dr. Brodie says. "It's better than an enema, which is merely a lower bowel cleanse, as opposed to a colonic which is a thorough cleanse of the entire bowel. It's similar to comparing the diagnostic efficacy of a sigmoid-oscopy of the short end of the bowel to a colonoscopy which takes in the whole bowel. An enema only goes so far. Colon hydrotherapy is the best cleansing and detoxifier for the gastrointestinal tract that anybody would want. I do promote its use."

CANCER AND THE PARASITE

Hulda Regeher Clark, Ph.D., ND, in her book, *The Cure for All Cancers*, says that all cancers are from solvent contaminates and parasites. I encourage you to read this book, but I will warn you, your head will spin from how many pollutants there are and their sources. She maintains that contaminants are contributing factors, but she states that the true cause is certain parasites. She states that each cancer is associated with a certain type of parasite.

BLOOD AND MONEY

The American public is being sold a bill of goods about cancer … Today the press releases coming out of the National Cancer Institute have all the honesty of the Pentagon.

– Dr. James Watson, Nobel Prize winner

The cancer industry is conservatively estimated to be worth an annual $50 to $75 billion, including treatment and research.

Cancer's Annual Treatment Costs (U.S.)

breast: $6.6. billion   *uterine:* $1.6 billion

colorectal: $6.5 billion   *melanoma:* $1.1 billion

lung: $5 billion   *leukemia:* $1.1 billion

prostate: $4.7 billion   *kidney:* $1 billion

bladder: $2.2 billion

ovarian, stomach, pancreatic, cervical: $610 million to $1 billion each

– *An Alternative Medicine Definitive Guide to Cancer*, 1997

A noted cancer specialist in Boston said he believed that if some simple and inexpensive replacement for chemotherapy as treatment of cancer were found tomorrow, all U.S. medical schools would teeter on the verge of bankruptcy. Oncology is integral to hospital revenues. The medical specialty of cancer treatment averages $50,000 to $75,000 per person per cancer, and that cost is rising. Cancer equals big money.

FALSE SECURITY

According to the medical journal *Acta Cytologica*, "False negatives are common in pap smears, occurring in about 30% of all cases." The error rate for cervical cancer may be as high as 50%. A woman may have several false negative pap tests in a row before falling ill and finding out that she has actually developed cervical cancer (Diamond, et al, 1997). As with most cancers we are at the mercy of conventional cancer screening which detects cancer in its later stages of development. True to the theme of this book, prevention is our optimal goal, and damage control after the disease is present is—in my opinion —just not acceptable. Detecting cancer in its earliest stages is imperative to increasing chances of survival for yourself and your loved one.

INFRARED THERMOGRAPHY SCANNING

Thermography is the most common term used to describe the procedure of thermal (heat) imaging. In simplest terms, thermography means "picture of heat." Infrared full body scanning is a totally safe and painless diagnostic imaging procedure that uses no radiation, injections, or other invasive procedures. Using technology developed by NASA and the aerospace sciences, HealthScan employs sophisticated infrared cameras and computer systems to scan the surface of the body for infrared thermal (heat) abnormalities. Abnormal patterns of heat are produced when dysfunctional systems and internal organs send nervous system signals to the surface of the body.

Thermography scanning provides patients with an early warning system. Unlike other forms of imaging that detect structural changes such as a tumor, infrared body scanning looks at the body's subtle chemical and nervous system changes. These neurochemical signals are sent far in advance of a build-up of cells large enough to be seen on a CT scan or MRI. Thermography has the ability to warn you 10 years in advance of any symptoms of a possible health problem.

THERMOGRAPHY IN BREAST CANCER PREVENTION

There are many current ideas and arguments on the subject of breast cancer. However, there are certain facts we know:

◆ Early detection holds the key to survival—especially if we can identify women who have high-risk pre-cancerous infrared imaging (breast thermography) markers.

◆ Mortality rates will go unchanged if earlier detection methods are not employed.

◆ There is currently no single test or procedure that is solely adequate for cancer screening.

◆ To minimize risk, keep the obvious risk factors under control and maintain a healthy diet and lifestyle.

◆ Thermography and mammography are complementary procedures; one test does not replace the other. When digital infrared imaging (thermography) is combined with mammography, a 61% increase in survival rate is realized.

◆ A multimodal (multiple testing) approach needs to be taken if thorough early detection is to be realized. If treated in the earliest detected stages, breast cancer cure rates greater than 95% are possible.

Since the prevention of breast cancer has not become a reality yet, efforts must be directed at extremely early detection. As the earliest known warning system, breast thermography gives a woman the chance to carefully monitor possible changes in the pre-cancerous process. In many cases, breast thermography has the ability to offer this warning *up to 8 to 10 years before a tumor can be detected by any other method.*

Therefore, in the absence of other positive tests, an abnormal infrared image gives a woman an early warning that a pathological process may be occurring. By maintaining close monitoring of her breast health with serial infrared imaging, self–breast exams, clinical examinations, and other tests, a woman has a much better chance of detecting cancer at its early stage and preventing invasive tumor growth.

Women with a family history are definitely at greater risk, but 75% of women who get breast cancer have no family history of the disease. If discovered, certain thermographic risk markers can warn a woman that she needs to be vigilant in monitoring her breast health.

The greatest single risk factor for breast cancer is lifetime exposure of the breasts to estrogen. Breast thermography plays a significant role in prevention by warning women if they have estrogen dominant activation of their breasts.

Approximately ⅓ of all breast cancers occur in women under age 45. This is the most common cancer in women in this age group. Breast cancers in younger women are usually more aggressive and have poorer survival rates. Breast thermography offers women under 40 a sensitive, non-invasive (no radiation and painless) method of monitoring their breast health beginning with baseline screening at age 20.

Unlike after-the-fact detection technologies (which find a cancerous tumor that is already there)—such as mammography, MRI, CT, ultrasound, and PET scans—breast thermography can give warning signals far in advance of an invasive tumor growth. Breast thermography offers a great deal of hope for the prevention of breast cancer and the future survival of women.

I have used thermography in the context of determining imbalances in the body that may result in cancer, but infrared thermography screening is also used for early detection of many physical imbalances that may result in impending disease. Infrared imaging is FDA-approved as an adjunctive diagnostic procedure.

This information on infrared thermography scanning was provided by the president of the International Academy of Clinical Thermology and clinical director of the Pacific Chiropractic and Research Center: William C. Amalu, DC, DABCT, DIACT, FIACT. Contact information for this life-saving screening is provided in the Resource Guide in Chapter 24.

DON'T SHOOT THE MESSENGER

If a patient dies of cancer without being informed that there were alternative treatment methods to those of established medical opinion, I believe it would be appropriate for his survivors to sue the doctors who failed to inform him.

— Robert C. Atkins, MD, *Nutrition Breakthrough*

I have strong feelings surrounding the subject of cancer. I lost both of my parents to this disease: my precious mother 26 years ago to breast cancer, and my father last year at age 70 to colon cancer. I have also witnessed the biased (profit-based) stance of national organizations that purport to lobby on the public's behalf. Whether it is the political, billion-dollar industry of cancer or the minimal regulation of the grocery store shelves, I have brought you information that may go against everything you have heard about cancer and its prevention.

My vested interest in the subject of cancer, both professionally and personally, has led me to some very controversial information. My intention is not to get too political here, but I feel passionately that this information must be brought to light and taken with extreme seriousness. Anything less than that, I feel, would be professionally irresponsible on my part.

I have referenced many books, journals, and documented resources that speak to the political aspect of cancer prevention and to alternative treatments. Please don't think for one minute that the subject of cancer is not highly political. I call cancer the subject of "blood and money." I encourage you to educate yourself and find out what's being said by these experts who have been out there on the political battlefield trying to expose the truth about national cancer agencies. I can only give you an overview on cancer in this book; I could not possibly give this subject full justice. I will leave that to those who have researched and gone head to head with the national agencies, in an effort to expose the truth to the public.

IF YOU OR A LOVED ONE HAVE CANCER

An important goal of this book is to illuminate the dark fact that most of what you have heard over your lifetime about cancer treatments is not the truth. At the very least, you have received an incomplete picture. If you believe the propaganda you have been fed and you develop cancer, it can cost you your life.

— An Alternative Medicine Definitive Guide to Cancer

I could not have said it better. Be informed. If you or a family member are facing the crisis of cancer, become an information sleuth. Read everything you can about your alternatives and choices. Cancer statistics being what they are (1 out of 3 people will get cancer), someone you know intimately in your lifetime will most likely be dealing with this life-challenging issue. If you have armed yourself with knowledge, you can make a decision from a position of power—not from fear and panic. (Please refer to Chapter 24, "Resource Guide," for alternative cancer prevention and treatment.)

In Loving Memory

Mother, it is so confusing for me now.
I want you to know me as a woman.
Yet, I want so much for you to hold me
and stroke my hair like you did when I was a little girl.
When death took you from my life,
I was still such a child.
Mother, there are so many times that I have needed you
and wanted just to talk with you.
Mother, I want so much for you to know my sons.
I wish you could cherish as I do
how caring and sensitive Brandon has become
and how mischievous and loving Christopher is
with that wide-eyed look of his.
Mother, if I could give a year of my life
just to hold you and see you again—
even for just a moment—I would freely give it.
Mother, I just want you to know how much I love
and miss you ...

– Loree

This chapter on cancer is dedicated to my mother Alice, who lost her life to this disease.

CHAPTER 10

■ ■ ■ ■ ■ ■ ■ ■ ■ ■

The Art of the Fart: Fluffy Floaters, Stinky Sinkies, and Other Medical Jargon

Have you ever come across absolute jewels of humor that really hit you between the eyes? Even though I am serious about these medical terms and jargon there is also the lighter side of poop! The last place I expected to find a sense of humor about the dreaded and embarrassing subject of, er, well, you know ... passing ... um ... "gas," was in a medical diagnostic textbook, the *Merck Manual*. But, lo and behold, an alert Dr. Ramsey, with a passion for humorous "tidbits," forwarded me this noteworthy information to pass (no pun intended) on to you, my readers. Of course, they use the technical term "flatulence" but you probably know it as "farting." You will see that there is a real art to "passing gas" or "farting."

Flatulence: among those who are flatulent, the quantity and frequency of gas passage shows great variability. As with bowel frequency, a person who complains of flatulence often has a misconception of what is normal. In a study of 8 normal men aged 25 to 35 years, the average number of gas passages was 4 to 13 in one day, with an upper limit of 21 per day, which overlapped with many persons who complained of excess flatus. On the other hand, one study noted a person who expelled gas as often as 141 times daily, including 70 passages in one 4-hour period. Hence, objectively recording flatus ... should be the first step in evaluating a complaint of excessive flatulence.

This symptom, which can cause great psychosocial distress, is unofficially described according to its silent characteristics:

◆ *The "slider" (crowded elevator type), which is released slowly and noiselessly, sometimes with a devastating effect.*

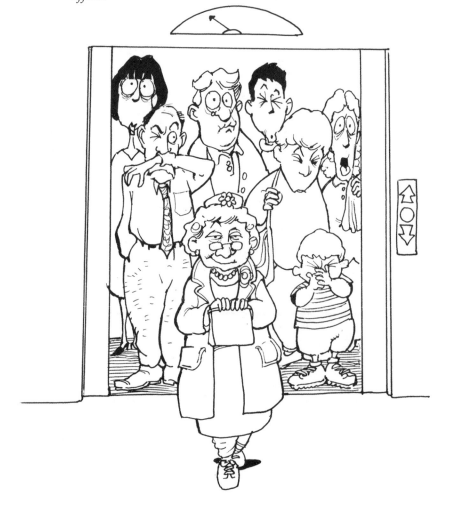

- *The open sphincter or "pooh" type, which is said to be of higher temperature and more aromatic.*

- *The staccato or drumbeat type pleasantly passed in privacy.*

- *The "bark" type (described as a personal communication) is characterized by a sharp exclamatory eruption that effectively interrupts (and often concludes) conversation. Aromaticity is not a prominent feature. Rarely, this usual distressing symptom has been an advantage, as with a Frenchman referred to as "Le Petomanc," who became affluent as an effluent performer who played tunes with the gas from his rectum on the Moulin Rouge stage.*

– Merck, 1997

TYPES OF CONSTIPATION

Atonic bowel. This is primarily a condition of the elderly, or someone confined to bed rest. Feces accumulate because the colon does not respond to the usual stimuli promoting evacuation, or accessory stimuli such as nutrition and exercise. This condition can occur in a person who disregards the normal urge to defecate, which results in diminishing or dulled rectal sensitivity to this sensation. This condition can be precipitated by prolonged dependence on laxatives. I have seen this condition in many people who have been on a heavy diet of refined carbohydrates.

Ballooning (of the colon). This occurs as a consequence of backed-up feces. For various reasons, feces can accumulate and stretch the bowel wall into enormous proportions. Adhesions, spasms, or colitis can cause this narrowing condition. When ballooning occurs, constipation can become quite severe and painful, and have a damaging effect upon the bowel structure and function.

Constipation. This condition generally develops as a result of unwise eating habits. Constipation is an undue and habitual delay in the evacuation of fecal waste from the large intestine. In order to determine the degree of constipation, we must know the transit time of material as it passes through the alimentary tract.

Diarrhea. This condition is characterized by the frequent passage of watery stools. The most common causes of diarrhea are viruses, food poisoning, parasites such as giardia, anxiety and nervousness, and reactions to food, alcohol, or medications. Other symptoms accompanying diarrhea that warrant medical attention include severe abdominal pain, confusion, unresponsiveness, or dizziness while standing.

Spastic constipation. Spasms of the large intestine interfere with peristalsis (wave motion that moves fecal matter), and delay evacuation of waste material.

OTHER BOWEL AND MEDICAL CONDITIONS

Adhesions (in the colon). These are caused by inflammations and irritations to the bowel wall. When the mucus membrane breaks down, tissue becomes exposed, open, and irritated. The raw surfaces begin to stick together as the result of a glue-like substance secreted from the tissue. This is a serious condition and requires delicate treatment to correct.

Inflammatory bowel disease. There are two types: ulcerative colitis and Chrohn's disease. Ulcerative colitis is a chronic inflammation of the mucous lining of the colon (large intestine) and the rectum. Raw, inflamed ulcers and small abscesses develop and, as a reaction, the colon tries to empty itself with great frequency, thus causing bloody diarrhea and left-sided pain.

Chrohn's disease. Another chronic inflammation, this condition can occur anywhere in the intestinal system but usually develops in the final section of the small intestine called the ileum. The inflammation appears as patches that seem to grow and spread. The patches can heal, but they leave scar tissue that thickens the intestinal wall and narrows the passageway. The symptoms are similar to ulcerated colitis, but with less diarrhea and more pain centered on the right side. Severe cases can involve bloody diarrhea, joint pain, fever, weight loss, and malnourishment.

Colon (colorectal) cancer. Either form of inflammatory bowel disease is associated with an increased risk of colon cancer according to Andrew Gaeddert, author of *Digestive Disorders* (1998). (Also see Chapter 9 on cancer.)

Colitis. This irritable bowel condition is strongly associated with psychological distress. Our emotions can upset the delicate processes in the body.

Colostomy. The large intestine is rerouted to a hole in the abdomen and emptied into a bag or pouch carried on the side of the patient.

Diverticulosis/diverticulitis. In this condition, diverticula — small pouches of intestinal lining — protrude inward from the large intestine. Known as diverticulosis, this affects 70% of the population between the ages of 40 and 70.

Gastritis. An inflammation of the stomach lining, this condition's main symptom is upper abdominal discomfort. Nausea, vomiting, and diarrhea may also be evident. In otherwise asymptomatic cases, gastric bleeding may be present and is characterized by blood in the vomit, or by black tarry stools. This is a serious condition usually requiring hospitalization.

Gastroesophageal reflux. Heartburn, with or without regurgitation of gastric contents into the mouth, is this condition's most prominent symptom. This disorder may also be experienced as a sour taste in the mouth or can involve burning pain in the upper abdomen and the middle chest. The acidic contents of the stomach flow back into the esophagus, causing inflammation. If you experience difficulty swallowing, or it feels like food is getting stuck on the way down, please see your physician immediately, since these signs may signal formation of esophageal cancer.

Hemorrhoids. Half or more of the adult population develops hemorrhoids. Hemorrhoids are literally varicose veins in the anus. They can lead to rectal pain, bleeding, and itching, or they can be relatively symptomless. The veins become swollen due to increased pressure inside them. They are common in pregnant women from the pressure of the fetus. Usually this situation is a result of persistent straining from body waste in the rectum. Fissures and cracks in the skin around the anus can also form. Bleeding from the rectum can also signal rectal cancer or polyps, so medical diagnosis is a must if you have these symptoms.

Hiatal hernia. In this condition a part of the stomach protrudes upward into the chest through an opening in the diaphragm. It tends to occur in obese persons, especially upper-middle-aged people, and in smokers. Most patients are asymptomatic (exhibiting no symptoms), but in some people spasms of the esophagus can result in acid reflux and bloating after meals. *The Merck Manual* (1997) states that x-rays usually demonstrate hiatal hernia. Many chiropractors and alternative health practitioners have techniques to help relieve hiatal hernia.

Intestinal obstruction. The partial or complete blockage of either the small intestine or the colon can be indicated by abdominal distention, spasms or cramping of the mid-abdomen, vomiting, and the inability to pass feces or intestinal gas. This can be a serious situation and can lead to a life-threatening condition; consult a physician immediately. Medical tests, such as x-ray, sigmoidoscopy, or colonoscopy, are conducted to assess the location of the obstruction. This delay in evacuation of feces is due to an obstruction in the intestine due to tumor, adhesions, etc.

Indigestion. This term covers many symptoms commonly experienced after eating, such as discomfort caused by a feeling of fullness in the upper abdomen, nausea, heartburn, and accompanied bloating.

Irritable bowel syndrome (IBS). This condition, which includes spastic colon, spastic colitis, mucous colitis, nervous stomach, and nervous diarrhea, is the #1 digestive disease in the United States, with over 30 million sufferers. It is estimated that up to 22% of the U.S. population has IBS, either occasionally or persistently. There are estimates that this condition is the second most common reason for absence from work or school. Poor diet and emotionally stressful situations usually trigger IBS. Despite this, IBS is actually one of the more treatable digestive conditions, responding well to exercise, stress reduction, and dietary modification.

Leaky gut syndrome. Leaky gut is a condition in which the mucosal lining of the intestinal tract becomes porous and irritated. Under normal conditions this intestinal mucosa allows essential nutrients (in the form of amino acids from digested foods) to pass through it and into the bloodstream. Simultaneously, this lining presents a physical and immunological barrier to the absorption of most large undigested food particles, intestinal toxins, parasites, and candida albicans (yeast). This lining acts like a traffic light, allowing nutrients to pass, while preventing unwanted food and toxins from getting through. Over time, the breakdown in this intestinal mucosa may result in the absorption of unwanted particles, toxins, parasites, and candida into the bloodstream. The end result is a weakened immune system, digestive disorder, and eventually chronic and autoimmune disease.

Megacolon. There are two types of megacolon:

◆ *Congenital megacolon (Hirchsprung's disease).* Due to the lack of normal nerve plexus (innervation) in the wall of the colon, feces accumulate before the diseased area, causing massive dilation of the bowel. Involves rectosigmoid area usually, but may involve the entire colon.

◆ *Acquired megacolon.* In contrast to the congenital type, the rectum is also distended and full of feces in the acquired condition. The colon also gradually becomes distended. This condition is seen in the mentally retarded or psychotic children who deny the urge to defecate.

Peptic ulcers. Raw areas affecting either the stomach or the upper part of the small intestine are involved. The stomach and upper intestine have specialized linings that normally resist digestion by acid or pepsin. Peptic ulcers can result when acids damage the lining of the stomach and intestinal linings. A burning pain or gnawing ache is felt just below the breastbone when acid invades these raw gastric ulcers. Please see your gastroenterologist if you feel ulcers are present because they can have fatal consequences, especially if there is a perforation of the organ wall into the abdominal cavity. One sign of this is black, tarry stools.

Polyps. These mushroom-like growths inside the colon wall can be related to cancer.

Prolapses. This condition involves a falling or downward displacement of the transverse colon. Pressure from the displaced transverse colon can seriously affect the organs below, such as the uterus, bladder, or prostate.

Rectal fissures. These are ulcerations of the skin of the anal canal that are actually longitudinal cracks in the skin. An acute fissure occurs as a result of stretching of the tissue and possibly from the trauma of a hard or large stool passing through the area.

Stricture. A narrowing of the intestinal wall, this condition usually is a result of Chrohn's disease or colitis.

Tumors. Both benign and malignant tumors may occur in all positions of the bowel, but their incidence varies greatly from one area to another. Malignant tumors are uncommon in the small bowel, representing only 1% of all tumors of the alimentary tract.

The Perfect Stool
by Robert M. Charm

Sitting on the stool committee of our local hospital
one day I did see (sitting directly behind me)
and down a little—round and firmly soft.
An easy push, odor and occult blood-free.
An easy wipe—one or two (rarely three)—
the end result of healthy food
high in fiber and low in fat and time to sit,
to sat, to beget: so get with it.
Produce the perfect stool!
Don't fight it. Don't be a fool.
Prevent the "piles" of trouble caused by
diverticulitis and polyps and cancer
and appendicitis. The best way to insure
against the "rrhoids" is not Lloyd's
of London. Lordy no!
Do your duty every day, one or two (or maybe three).
Don't wait, don't regurge; heed the urge. Release.

Used with permission by Robert M. Charm, MD,
specialist in gastroenterology and internal medicine

FLUFFY FLOATERS OR STINKY SINKIES

My personal thanks to Amanda Gore, an Australian professional speaker, whose creative description of fluffy floaters and stinky sinkies graces this book for all of us to enjoy. I always appreciate the poop-related humor of others.

What Is Your Type of Poop?

◆ *Rock hard stools.* Constipation, diets low in roughage and/or water, sedentary individuals, persons who ignore body signals for pooping.

◆ *Poorly formed stools.* Diarrhea, diets with too much roughage, colon with too little muscle tone, poor food combinations, and/or food allergies.

◆ *Thin or "ribbon" stools.* Spasms or obstructions anyplace from the descending colon through the anal passage, tightly coiled sigmoid colon, enlarged prostate.

◆ *Fluffy floaters (floating stools).* Can be high-fat diets, persons with poor absorption or digestion of fats, high mucus conditions.

◆ *Stinky sinkies (foul-smelling stools).* Poor digestion, poor food combinations, increased colon transit times, wrong bacteria in the colon.

◆ *Mucous stools.* Irritated colon, ulcerative colitis, diets high in mucus-producing foods (milk, cheese, etc.), food allergies or sensitivities.

What Color Is Your Poop?

◆ *Red blood in stools.* Can be from hemorrhoids, or bleeding in lower intestinal tract.

◆ *Black stools.* Can indicate bleeding in stomach or small intestines; ingestion of too much iron, certain berries, or beets.

Activated charcoal and hydrated bentonite can cause the stools to be dark gray or black in color.

♦ *Green stools.* Can indicate problems with the production and/or conversion of bile, or too much chlorophyll.

♦ *Light-colored stools.* Can indicate insufficient bile production, or gall bladder obstructions.

♦ *Bright yellow stools.* Vegetarian, overexcretion of bile, acidity in the bowel.

♦ *Gray or white stools.* Can mean malfunction of liver, or gallbladder can be totally blocked.

What does "healthy poop" look like? The answer surprises most people. A truly healthy individual with a truly healthy colon, eating the foods we are meant to eat, produces a stool that is typically a medium brown color, 1 to 1½ inches in diameter, many inches long, well formed, almost odorless, and that moves through the anal canal without any straining. You might see such a stool from young children, but most adults rarely have such stools on a regular basis. Age, inadequate diet, lack of exercise, too much stress, and unfavorable genetics—to name a few causes—all have their degenerative effects. The stools produced just aren't what they used to be. The aforementioned are examples of conditions and some possible causes of a certain type of stool.

DIAGNOSTIC PROCEDURES

The following are descriptions of the leading diagnostic procedures to evaluate the full colon (colonoscopy), and the sigmoid, or lower colon (sigmoidoscopy), as well as the barium enema as described by the *Merck Manual.*

Colonoscopy. Used to further evaluate an abnormality seen on barium enemas; to determine the source of occult or gastrointestinal bleeding or unexplained (microcytic) anemia; to evaluate pre- or post-operatively for other lesions in patients with colonic cancer; to determine the extent of inflammatory bowel disease. After a rectal examination, the colonoscope is gently inserted through the anal sphincter into the rectum. Under direct visualization, air is infused and the instrument is manipulated through the colon to the cecum. The patient may experience cramp-like discomfort that may be relieved by aspiration of the air, or rotation or retraction of the tube, or may need additional medication. Diagnostic evaluation is performed using visualization of structures, photograph, and obtaining brushings or biopsy of abnormal structures. This test is recommended every 10 years.

Sigmoidoscopy. Used to examine the patient with symptoms referable to the rectum or anus (e.g., bright rectal bleeding, discharge protrusions, pain); to evaluate a lesion known to be within reach of the instrument; to evaluate the rectum or sigmoid colon before anorectal surgery; to evaluate the rectum in any patient in whom a barium enema is indicated (barium enema does not adequately visualize this area). After the rectal examination, the perianal area is examined, and the lubricated instrument is gently inserted 3 to 4 cm past the anal sphincter for direct vision. This test is recommended every 5 years in conjunction with an annual stool test.

Barium enema. In a contrast barium enema, a technician coats the inside of the intestine with metallic dye and fills the colon full of air. Then an x-ray of the large intestine is taken, allowing doctors to see the outline of most abnormal growths. Provided the colon is clear, a barium enema should be repeated every 5 to 10 years.

Please do not use any of these descriptions in this chapter to self-diagnose. Consult your physician if there is any significant change in the nature of your stools or bowel habits. Over the years I have had many clients with rectal bleeding and I always encourage them to go in for medical testing. It can be something as benign as internal fissures, but you do not want to take that chance. Bleeding can also be a sign of cancer. If you have any—I mean any—bleeding from the bowel or in your stool, run (do not walk) to your doctor of internal medicine to have the appropriate testing for a diagnosis.

Once Upon a Colon
by Robert M. Charm

Once upon a colon
I did see
via colonoscopy
a healthy tube of colon pink
a conduit so fit
cleaned carefully of . . . it;
polyp, cancer, divertic-free
IBS, spastic colitis or IBD*
So you be smart
and come see me:
Yes—it's time for your colonoscopy.

* Inflammatory bowel disease

Used with permission by Robert M. Charm, MD,
specialist in gastroenterology and internal medicine

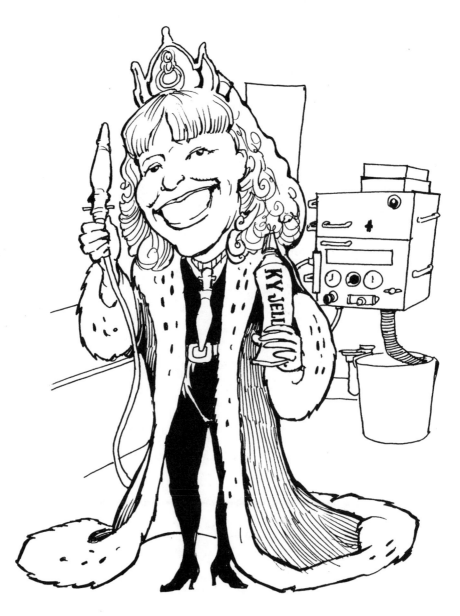

The Colonic Queen™

CHAPTER 11

■ ■ ■ ■ ■ ■ ■ ■ ■ ■

You Want to Put Water WHERE?

HISTORY OF COLON CLEANSING

Colon hydrotherapy is the pathway to vibrant health! In one form or another, cleansing of the large intestine (bowel or colon) has been practiced since 1500 B.C. Colon lavage was first recorded in the ancient Egyptian document, *Ebers Papyrus*, which dealt with the practice of medicine. These enemas were described as the infusion of aqueous (water) substances into the large intestine (bowel or colon) through the anus. Hippocrates (4th and 5th century B.C. recorded using enemas for fever therapy. Pare, in 1600 A.D., offered the first recognized distinction between colon irrigation and the popular enema therapy of that age.

Since the turn of the century, colon hydrotherapy has alternated between periods of popularity and periods of skepticism. This ambivalence, resulting from untrained and unskilled practitioners performing this valuable therapy, has undermined its growth. In the early 1900s popular physicians such as James W. Wiltsie, MD, and Joseph E.G. Waddington, MD, were proponents of colon hydrotherapy. They placed great value on the therapeutic benefits of this modality. With regard to the lack of priority given the colon by many physicians, Dr. Wiltsie stated: "Our knowledge of the normal and abnormal physiology of the colon, and of its pathology and management, has not kept pace with that of many organs and systems of the body. As long as we continue to assume that the colon will take care of itself, just that long will we remain in complete ignorance of perhaps the most important source of ill health in the whole body."

Joseph E. G. Waddington, MD, said: "Abnormal functioning of the intestinal canal is the precursor of much ill health, especially of chronic disease conditions. Restoration of physiologic intestinal elimination is often the first, but too-often ignored, important preliminary to eventual restoration of the health in general."

Unfortunately, with misunderstandings and preconceived ideas, controversy continues to surround colon hydrotherapy. Historically, we recognize two unequivocal conclusions. First, there is something of value to this modality or it would have been conclusively withdrawn. Second, because of lack of professional control and study, colon hydrotherapy never received the attention and recognition it justly deserves.

With today's modern technological advancements in colon hydrotherapy instrumentation, particularly with regard to safety, along with educated and skilled hydrotherapists, colon hydrotherapy has become a valuable adjunctive modality to physicians in treating disease. Yet colon hydrotherapy is still misunderstood in this enlightened era. As recently as February 2000, articles in popular magazines continue to tout the dangers of colon hydrotherapy.

Combined with sound nutrition, exercise, and a positive mental and spiritual outlook, colon hydrotherapy can play an integral role in achieving optimal and vibrant health.

WHAT IS COLON HYDROTHERAPY?

One of the most important and effective ways to cleanse the colon is through colon hydrotherapy, also known as colonics. Colon hydrotherapy is clean and relaxing. A soothing flow of filtered, temperature-controlled water gently circulates throughout the colon, coaxing your body to release the digested toxins and waste that may have built up inside. Colon hydrotherapy is an ancient, time-honored, gentle water cleansing of the colon, by way of a sterile, disposable rectal tube or speculum. Water in—fecal matter flushed out.

A colonic machine is attached to a wall and directly linked to the sewer system. A clear, contained tube (no smell or odor) allows viewing of the waste material before it goes into the sewer system. A colonic is facilitated by a trained colon hydrotherapist who administers and regulates the flow of water into the bowel. Most clients say that a colonic is more comfortable than they had first imagined. Other modalities that may also be used during a colonic are reflexology on the feet, massage of lymphatic areas, heat lamp treatment, and aromatherapy oils to aid the body in releasing toxins. The treatment lasts about 45 to 60 minutes.

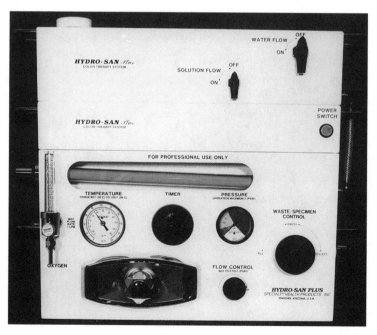

Hydro-San Plus colonic machine

FREQUENTLY ASKED QUESTIONS

I would like to address some of the most common asked questions clients have about colon hydrotherapy.

Is colon therapy embarrassing?

After the gentle insertion of a small tube into the rectum, rubber tubing carries the water in and wastes out in a gently pressurized system. No mess, no fuss, no odor—in fact, a very relaxing experience. Except for the insertion of the tube you are completely covered during the entire procedure.

Is the procedure painful?

Rarely. Sometimes during the procedure the muscles of the colon contract suddenly, expelling considerable liquid and waste into the rectum. The contraction may feel like cramping or gas with pressure in the rectum. Most of the process is mild and gentle with a wonderfully light and empty feeling afterwards.

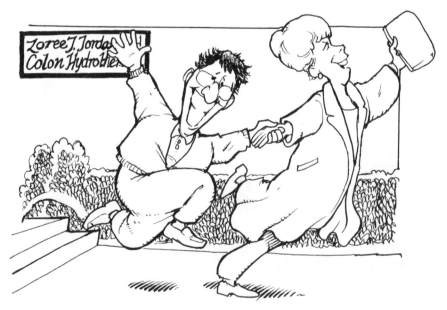

After the colonic

Will one cleansing completely empty the colon?

Almost never. Many of us have 10 or more pounds of impacted feces in our colon. This is hardened, rubbery material and substantial work must be done to remove it. One cleansing removes some; the second, more. Your personal objectives will determine how many you may wish to have.

Does colon therapy wash away all bacteria, even the good?

The helpful bacteria can only live in an acidic environment, whereas the harmful ones thrive in an alkaline environment. Most people, due to years of improper eating, lack of exercise, and poor elimination, have an alkaline colon. So it *is* helpful to flush away the bacteria in an alkaline colon. The great benefit of the cleansing program is to change the environment from alkaline to acid.

Is the procedure safe and sanitary?

With the use of high-tech disposable apparatus, the equipment is made "new" every session. There is total hygienic safety, superior even to sterilization.

What other benefits may I expect from colon hydrotherapy?

Colon hydrotherapy is not a cure, but a valuable procedure used to assist the body with a wide variety of colon-related conditions. By re-toning the bowel wall and improving colon functions, the entire body is able to function more efficiently.

Common effects are sinus drainage, a loosening of mucous in the lungs, improved range of motion, skin tightening, feeling younger, clearing up of acne and skin conditions, improved posture, abdomen softening and shrinking, a relief from headaches, less fatigue, and improved bowel function. Colon hydrotherapy works to soothe and tone the colon, helping it to eliminate more efficiently. The function as a whole reduces the burden on other organs and the lymphatic system. The main benefit received from releasing the old toxic waste is that we remove the #1 source of disease in the body. The bowel then works more efficiently in eliminating waste, and nutrient absorption is improved.

Will laxatives or enemas accomplish the same results?

Using an enema you are missing about 4 feet of the colon. During a colonic the water goes all the way through 5 feet of the colon or bowel to the ileocecal valve (this is where the small and large intestine meet). Laxatives are an irritant, causing the body to produce a thin, watery substance that goes through the colon and leaves behind impacted toxins and waste on the walls of the colon. Laxatives can also become very habit-forming.

Why can't I just take an enema instead of a colonic?

J. Waddington, MD, says there is no resemblance of one to the other, except that both proceed with water in the rectum. Enemas use single, high-volume, pressurized fills, sometimes fatiguing the colon. Colon hydrotherapy, on the other hand, involves repeated inflow and outflow of filtered, temperature-controlled water, to slowly dissolve accumulated toxic material. This gently repeated process replaces the need for pressure. Less pressure is used than when "bearing down" during bowel movements. Colon hydrotherapy is far more effective and comfortable. Colonics also exercise the colon, weakened by poor bowel habits and burdensome foods. Unlike enemas, no strain is exerted on the anus, preventing aggravation to hemorrhoids.

Can one become dependent on it? Could the colon stop functioning on its own?

Colon hydrotherapy retrains the muscle of the bowel to regain strength. The bowel muscle is forced to work against the water, providing resistance much like a weight provides resistance against a muscle in bodybuilding. After the bowel has regained its strength, it works better on its own. I tell clients that colonics are like colon aerobics.

Won't I flush out all the good bacteria with a colonic?

If your bowel is toxic you have little or no good intestinal flora to begin with. As in gardening, if you do not prepare the soil and fertilize the ground, plants will not live. In the bowel we have to make the conditions favorable for bifidophilus and acidophilus cultures to populate in the colon. Removing toxic material and gases is the first step. Replenishing the good bacteria can be accomplished by oral supplementation and by adding bifidophilus as an additive after your colonic treatment. Your colon hydrotherapist can show you how to give yourself an implant at home after a colonic treatment.

EXTERNAL CLEANSING VITAL TO SUCCESS OF DETOXIFICATION

A colonic is critically important during a cleansing and detoxification program because it keeps the body from reabsorbing toxins back into the body. Let me explain. As you are taking herbs and supplements to detoxify your body you can be overloaded with releasing toxins. If these increased toxins are not effectively removed from the body quickly via the bowel with colonics, they will be reabsorbed into the bloodstream and carried throughout the whole body. This can cause discomforts such as malaise, nausea, headaches, joint and muscle aches, and foul-smelling breath. Detoxification and cleansing can cause some healing discomforts which we will discuss later when we talk about the healing crisis, but colonics will keep those discomforts to a minimum.

Colonics are nothing to be afraid of. Many people have said to me, "But they are unnatural." I typically respond, "But our diet has been unnatural, also."

DO I REALLY HAVE TO DO THIS?

Many clients have asked me if they can do cleansing without participating in external colon cleansing. I believe that

121

cleansing the bowel is essential for the reasons just stated (to limit the re-absorption of toxins) and for the success of a cleansing program. I am pretty non-negotiable on this. I would feel professionally irresponsible if I allowed someone to start a cleanse without knowing all the facts.

HOW TO USE THE COLEMA BOARD™ (HOME COLONIC UNIT)

1.   Assemble the board according to the instructions provided (sent with the board).

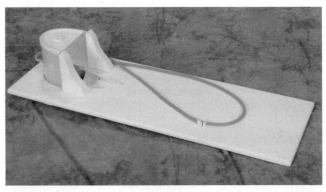

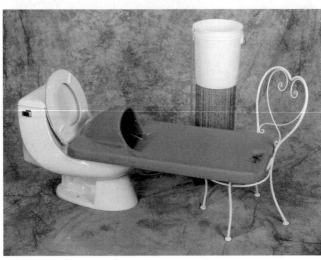

2. Fill a 5-gallon bucket with purified water (room temperature to body temperature is fine). There are a number of different things you can add to the water which are recommended. (Choose only one of the below additives per session.) Please do not use tap water, which can contain chlorine and microscopic organisms that will absorb into the body through the bowel.

Lemon juice. Add ¼ cup of strained lemon juice to 5 gallons of water.

Epsom salts. Add one tablespoon of Epsom salts to 5 gallons of water.

Garlic. Cut up 4 cloves of garlic and put in blender with 1 cup of water. Then add this to your large bucket of water. Great choice when fighting infection or parasitic infestation.

Coffee. Put 3 tablespoons of ground coffee (not instant or flavored) in a quart of water. Bring to a boil and simmer 15 minutes. Strain through strainer and add water to make 5 gallons. Coffee is excellent to stimulate the liver.

Bentonite. Add 1 cup of bentonite (montorillonite) to your 5-gallon bucket. This helps kill unfavorable bacteria in the colon.

3. After your colonic water is all set up, make sure to put an old kitchen colander (strainer) in the toilet. This will catch any hardened mucous and fecal matter. This will be proof of what wretched material is harbored in the colon.

4. Next, lubricate the thin plastic or stainless steel rectal tube for easy insertion into the rectum. Please do not share tubing with family members: everyone using the Colema Board *must have their own separate tubing.*

5. Make sure you put several towels on the board. The more, the better. The Colema Board can get quite hard without a soft cushion.

6. Make sure the water is about 2 feet above your body. You can lower or raise it a little to adjust the rate at which the water will enter your body. You will have to get suction in the hose before it will flow down. To do this, fill the plastic hose up with water and let some of it out. This will create suction. Then clamp it and put one end in the 5-gallon bucket.

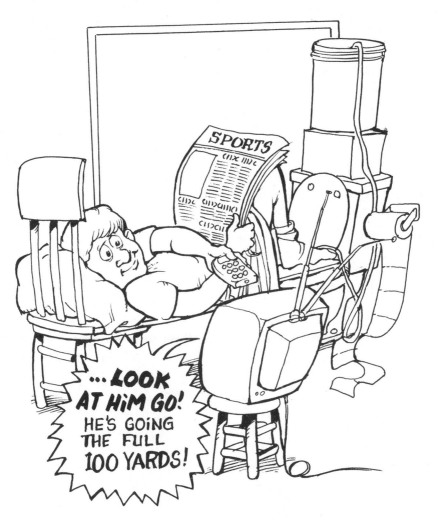

7. Do not try to hold too much water in the beginning. If you feel any pressure, then simply "let go" and the water will come pouring out directly into the toilet. The more you get used to taking home colonics, the more you will know exactly how much you can hold.

8. Try to massage your colon as much as you can. Start on the lower left and work your way around the colon. In many cases you will be able to hold more water if you just massage your colon a little and then let more water in.

9. Once you start using the Colema Board you should continue until your colon is clean. It is best not to start for just a few days and then drop the program. Only start if you can carry through for at least a month, and then continue on a regular basis.

10. Be sure to clean and sanitize immediately after each use. Use a strong antiseptic, but make sure it will not damage the tubing. Remember, do not share tubing with family members!

Some Advantages of the Colema Board

Do it yourself/privacy. With the Colema Board, you can give yourself a colonic treatment right in the privacy of your own home. You don't have to rely on anyone to give you a treatment. Many people are very uncomfortable about going to a colon hydrotherapist and being in a vulnerable position. Anybody in the family can use the board, from seven-year-olds up to someone in their 90s.

Lower financial investment. Outside of the initial cost of the Colema Board, there is no additional cost for each colonic treatment. If finances are an issue for you or your family, this is the way to go. Colonics can run from $60 to $95 per treatment. Note: A set of tubing will be required for every member of the family and this will be an additional purchase cost to the Colema Board.

Portable unit. The Colema Board is portable. You can easily use it in any hotel or motel. You can purchase a Colema Board that folds in the middle for easy transportation.

You see your results. One of the best advantages of using the Colema Board is that you can actually see the results. By using a simple kitchen colander, you can catch the results in the toilet and see and smell for yourself how much putrid matter came out of you. As I have said before there is no substitute for experience.

Relaxed atmosphere. With the home Colema Board, you can be totally relaxed while you are giving yourself a colonic. You are in your own familiar surroundings. I used to bring in music and light candles and just relax during my treatments.

You are in control. With the home Colema Board, you are in complete control of your treatment. Since you are controlling the water flow yourself, you know exactly how much water to let in and you know exactly when to let the water out. And you don't have to rely on someone else to receive a treatment.

DID YOU SAY ENEMA?
Instructions for a Complete Enema

Equipment needed:

♦ *Enema bag* (you can obtain this in any pharmacy) or an enema set-type bucket with a 22-foot flexible Dynaclamp. [Ordering information is in the Resource Guide (Chapter 24).] If I was going to give myself an enema this is what I would use.

♦ *A Davol colon tube.* This is a flexible red rubber tube, 18 to 30 inches long, that attaches to the hard plastic enema tip. It provides more safety and comfort than the standard attachment. These are available from medical supply stores and come in different sizes, denoted by their French number. This number designates the interior diameter of the tube; higher numbers indicate a larger diameter or the ability to pass more solution in a given time. Fr. #26 to Fr. #30 are standard sizes for average adults, Fr. #18 is used for young children, and the intermediate numbers are for ages in between.

♦ *K-Y jelly* for a lubricant. This is used to make insertion of the rectal tube easier and more comfortable.

♦ *A pad or heavy bath towel.* This is placed underneath the buttocks during the enema. You may obtain a "chuck" from the medical supply store. This is a pad that is absorbent on one side and plastic on the other side. This pad helps absorb any leakage.

Instructions:

1. For best results and your own comfort, the enema must be taken while lying down. Use a common enema bag, suspended no more than 18 to 24 inches above where the rectum will be receiving the water, so that the water pressure will not be too strong. The best place to give yourself an enema is in the bathtub or bathroom floor. Use purified water (since the colon absorbs the water back into the bloodstream), warmed to about 100°F.

2. Open the shutoff for a moment and allow enough water to flow to expel the air from the enema tubing. This helps to reduce cramping once you start the enema.

3. Lubricate the rectal nozzle generously and lubricate your anal area with the K-Y jelly for easier insertion.

4. Hang the enema bag or bucket on a hook 18 to 24 inches above the rectum.

5. Start by lying on your left side. Gently insert the rectal tubing 3 to 4 inches into the rectum. Open the shutoff valve and allow the solution to flow. At the first indication of discomfort stop the flow and wait a few moments. Remember to breathe,

and relax. When you feel pressure, like a bubble of gas in the splenic flexure under the left rib, turn onto your back, allowing the transverse colon to fill. After about half of the water has been introduced into the colon, clamp off the flow and, without withdrawing the rectal tube, slowly turn over onto your back and pull your knees up. Keep a hand on the rectal tube so it doesn't accidentally slip out. When you are in a comfortable position, release the shutoff and resume the enema. When you feel full, stop the water flow, remove the rectal tube, and turn onto your right side. Massage the hepatic flexure (below right rib cage) by jiggling it to open and let gravity move the water through from the transverse colon area all the way to the cecum (lower right side) if possible.

6. Remain in position and retain the solution for at least 5 minutes—preferably 10 to 15 minutes. Follow your urge to release whenever your body tells you.

7. Go to the toilet and expel the enema. An enema seldom comes out in a single movement so stay near the toilet for 30 to 60 minutes. After expelling the enemas, most people find it comfortable to lie on the bed, on their back, and rest for a while. If results are inadequate, repeat the enema.

8. Be sure to clean your equipment thoroughly. Rinse out the enema bag (because intestinal pressure can cause reflux, a backing up of solution and colon waste into the bag). Then refill the bag partway with water, reattach the tubing if disconnected, and allow the water to flow into the sink, rinsing out the tubing. Hang up to dry. An enema bag takes several days to thoroughly dry out, and should never be put away while even slightly wet.

9. Remove any traces of K-Y jelly from the rectal tube and properly sanitize your equipment. You can soak in a bleach solution: 1 part bleach to 4 parts pure water for one hour. Rinse thoroughly after soaking.

Final tips:

◆   Retaining the enema solution for a while before expelling can significantly contribute to better results. Try to retain the enema for 15 minutes if possible. It is sometimes uncomfortable, but the results are worth the effort. At least 5 minutes should be the absolute minimum. During this time the enema has time to work its way up into the upper recesses of the bowel, and dissolve the hard, caked fecal coating on the interior wall of the bowel.

◆   Last but not least, try to relax during this whole process. It will make the enema much more successful.

(Most enemas clean only up to the sigmoid flexure and rarely go past the splenic flexure where most of the toxins are being reabsorbed. That is why I recommend colonic irrigations or the Colema Board over enemas.)

RECTAL IMPLANTS

After the fecal matter has been removed and cleansed from the bowel you may give yourself an implant. A rectal implant is exactly what is says: an implant of solution into the rectum. A rectal implant can be used after a professional colonic, a Colema (home colonic), or an enema. One of the purposes of an implant is to replenish healthy intestinal flora, such as acidophilus or bifidophilus, into the colon. A rectal implant can also serve as a way of getting supplementation into the body through the porous colon wall. A few examples of this would be rectal implants of wheatgrass juice, shark cartilage, vitamin C, and garlic, to name just a few.

I prefer an enema bucket with a Dynaclamp to be used as a method of rectal implantation. Lie on your left side and slowly administer the implant solution. Remember to relax and breathe. Until you get used to holding an implant, you may only be able to hold it for a few minutes (5 minutes or so). The ultimate goal is to hold the solution in the rectum for a full 20 minutes. Whatever solution is not absorbed into the body (after maximum holding time is reached) can be released into the toilet. There are so many variations of supplements, please discuss your particular health issues with your health practitioner or colon hydrotherapist.

Some final tips from colon hydrotherapists to improve the function of your colon:

1. Learn proper food combinations. Eat 50 to 70% of your foods raw. They should be fresh, organic, and in season from your local area. Consume a wide variety, but eat smaller quantities. Drink half your weight in ounces of water daily: sip it, not with meals, either 1 or 1½ hours before meals or 2 hours after meals.

2. Chew your foods properly by slowing down while eating and by relaxing.

3. Reduce stress and tension by exercising daily and getting adequate sleep.

4. Avoid intestinal overloading by responding to the "call of nature" immediately.

FINAL THOUGHTS

In this chapter I wanted to present you with a variety of options and choices to assist you in cleansing and detoxifying your colon. Just as everyone drives a different car to suit their needs, likes, and dislikes, so it is with your choice of method for colon cleansing.

I personally do not like to take enemas and never have. I used the home colonic unit (Colema Board) with great success for years before starting my practice and having access to a colonic machine. However, many people have used enemas for years and wish to stay with that procedure. Everyone has their own preference. Many of my colonic clients have purchased the Colema Board to supplement their colonics with home care a few times a week.

If you choose to colon cleanse at home, be sure to secure privacy from the other members of your household. Relaxation is crucial to the overall success of releasing the bowels. If you need to hire a babysitter, then by all means hire one. Kids screaming and fighting outside the bathroom door will not be conducive to this healing process. As a mother, I speak from experience. Trust me on this one.

After selling my colon hydrotherapy practice (to devote my time to writing and professional speaking) I had a Hydro-san colon hydrotherapy machine installed in my home bathroom! Believe me, it is a conversation piece when company comes over. Am I devoted to colon cleansing, or what? But that's me. You might not be willing to spend $5,000 to have a colon hydrotherapy machine installed in your bathroom.

You are the only one who knows your financial status and personal lifestyle, and you will do what suits you and your family the best. You will make the right choice.

MEN WHO GET COLONICS AND THE WOMEN WHO LOVE THEM

I don't know why it is that men in general have a harder time with colon hydrotherapy. I can tell you I would have fared much better in the dating world as a beautician than as a colon hydrotherapist. I am now a patient of the dentist that I had previously worked for. While getting a dental exam, Dr. Eddie tells me, "Loree, date a guy five or six times and *then* tell him what your profession is." My response is, "No, if I tell him on the first date and he runs, then I have saved us both some time. This just weeds out the wimps right up front." A man once brought me *Everyone Poops*, a children's book, on our first date. Call me old-fashioned, but whatever happened to getting roses? I'm not trying to single men out ... but in all my years as a colon hydrotherapist men have been the most apprehensive.

It is not unusual for men to send in their wives or girl-friends first, before they will come in for treatment. I used to tease the women and ask, "If you come back alive then your husband will come in?"

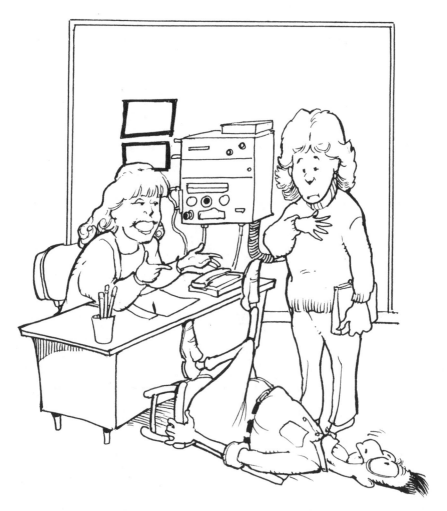

"Mrs. Perry, I just recommended that your husband have a series of colonics!"

We used to get some real laughs at how protective men are over their tushies. It must be a guy thing. I guess it is just not macho for a guy to wear a backless gown with a full view of his backside. Maybe because, as women, we are used to pregnancy, childbirth, pap smears etc., we seem to deal with these little embarrassing physical inconveniences with less apprehension. I just love it when male clients ask me if the slight cramping that can occur during a colonic hydrotherapy session is what it is like to experience childbirth. I just smile and tell them a little intestinal gas versus moving a huge baby down the birthing canal ... that is a real stretch (pun intended). How could a man even begin to understand childbirth, anyway?

Conversely, men as a rule seem to be more comfortable talking about their pooping habits and problems with gas. Men also seem to have fewer perceived problems with constipation than their female counterparts. Many women express the wish that they could poop like their husband or boyfriend. I tend to believe that this is partly due to our hormones. Also, women seem to feel stress (from working outside the home, raising children, housework etc.) more in their intestinal area. I am not saying men don't assist in housework and child-raising (I know men who do). It is just that women tend to feel (in their gut) more responsible for all these tasks simultaneously. The stress then takes its toll on us physically in the form, for example, of constipation.

It was stated at a Speaking for Women's Health conference in the Bay Area recently that women make 75% of all health care decisions. As women we have taken on the role of the family nurturer and, it seems, health care manager and advisor. It is our responsibility to be informed.

So ladies, hopefully you don't have to drag your men into the colon hydrotherapist's office kicking and screaming! We can support them with information, with our experiences, and by our example of how to improve our health through detoxification.

Some ladies, such as Ruth, will have to take drastic measures to help their husbands. Her husband David was completely resistant to colon cleansing. She had approached him many times with Dr. Bernard Jensen's book *Tissue Cleansing through Bowel Management* and the subject of colon cleansing; he just did not want to hear it. He thought all this stuff about colon cleansing was just a load of crap!

Ruth had heard me on one of the local radio shows promoting my new book. As a special promotion I was giving away my 90-minute audiotape, *Unleash the Power of Your Health,* free with every book order. She ordered the book and tape and also the Loree's Kick Butt bowel blaster products.

Ruth knew that there was no way she would get David to read my book as she had. So she devised a plan. On a drive to Santa Cruz and Monterey with her husband and their three kids—ages 17, 14, and 13—she hid my *Unleash the Power of Your Health* audio cassette tape into her purse. On the way to the beach she quietly listened to every CD the kids wanted. In Sync, you name it, she heard it. They had a great day on their day trip but on the way back she stated firmly that, since she quietly listened to their music, in return she wanted the whole family to listen to my audio tape. Fair is fair. Everyone whined and complained at first but they listened. Obviously they were a captive audience stuck in a car together; they had no choice, and it was a long walk home.

David had the most profound reaction. All of a sudden colon cleansing wasn't such a load of crap after all! After 90 minutes of hearing my voice hammer on him about yucky, clogged colons and parasites, he started to crack. When they got home David wanted Ruth to go to the health food store right away and get some colon cleansing products. He said he wanted to cleanse his colon immediately, if not sooner! Ruth told him she had ordered products from my office and they were in the mail. She also had ordered the Colema Board which he could use at home.

He has now used the Colema Board and has begun taking my bowel blaster drink. His wife told me that David is going to do the 7-day boot camp cleanse this very summer. Ruth has now sent my audio tape to Australia to some family members to motivate them also.

Their kids were also impacted by what they heard on my audio tape. Especially the part about the parasites. I have to tell you, those parasite stories are not for the faint at heart. The idea of worms crawling around in our intestines can get to the best of us. The two older children are going to embark on some colon cleansing this summer.

Okay let's recap ... David was a man that would not even discuss bowel cleansing and now he can't get his wife to help him cleanse fast enough. He is very conscious of proper food combining when he is eating and reminds his family. He keeps talking with his own mother, who unfortunately has the same attitude about this subject that he once had. He hasn't given up hope on his mother yet. Maybe he should take his mother on a drive to the beach with my audio tape. She may come home a changed woman. Or then again, she may cut him out of her will.

REAL MEN GET COLONICS

Okay, okay. I am not trying to give men a bad rap here. They are great clients and, I must say, usually the most entertaining. It is just getting those macho guys into the office and then into those backless gowns that seems to be the problem. If I told you all of the funny jokes and comments men come up with regarding the insertion of the speculum and this whole colon cleansing process, then this book would be X-rated. It is a good thing I have a sense of humor or I never would have survived all these years in this profession.

I once had a new male client in my office who was hysterically funny with all of his barbs and jokes about his vulnerability on my colonic table. He was so funny I could not resist a few jokes myself. His main concern seemed to be how he would know when he was "full of water," and would I know when to shut the water off? I looked at him calmly and said, "Well, you can usually tell your intestines are full when water shoots out your ears."

"Oh my God," he said.

I just smiled at him. When he realized I was kidding and giving him a dose of his own medicine, he relaxed. He had a great colonic session and felt wonderful when he left. In all seriousness, male clients make up about 30 to 40% of my practice, and they are a joy. Keep up the good work, guys!

CHAPTER 12

■ ■ ■ ■ ■ ■ ■ ■ ■ ■ ■

What Other Health Professionals Are Saying

The value of colon hydrotherapy is verified by medical professionals prescribing it. Portions of this chapter are reprinted with permission from the Townsend Letter for Doctors & Patients, August/September 2000 (#205/206) by Morton Walker, DPM.

COLON HYDROTHERAPY IS USUAL FOR THE PATIENTS OF W. JOHN DIAMOND, MD

For W. John Diamond, MD, medical director of the Triad Medical Center in Reno, Nevada, and co-author of that useful consumer text, *An Alternative Medicine Definitive Guide to Cancer*, colon hydrotherapy or high colonic irrigations are usual modalities to which he refers his patients. "For some patients with chronic constipation or extensive yeast problems, colon hydrotherapy works advantageously to get rid of the physical load of pathology in the gastrointestinal tract. This treatment stimulates the liver and gets rid of the debris that's sticking to the mucosa. The last time I referred my patient to take colon hydrotherapy was just yesterday. There's hardly a week that goes by which does not see me utilize this fabulous treatment for one or more patients. The colon hydrotherapist in this city of Reno is skilled and does a fine job.

"Let me describe a particular patient of mine who benefitted from colon hydrotherapy," says Dr. Diamond. "This woman at age forty-six has a long history of antibiotic usage for chronic sinusitis. She is a sugarholic to the extent that her food is totally carbohydrates with hardly any protein or fat. She exhibits a variety of symptoms including extreme fatigue, migraine headaches, irregular menses, chronic constipation, abdominal pain, and yeast growing in the bowel upon testing EAV (electroacupuncture according to Voll). Presence of the yeast was confirmed by stool culture and blood tests for yeast antibodies and skin testing.

"For such a complicated case, I tried every kind of treatment that was appropriate, but nothing did any good. The only program that gave this patient relief was colon hydrotherapy three times a week. It took me a month to get my patient stable, but finally the treatments' effect kicked in. The lady did get her bowel cleaned up; she's now experiencing normal stools and following a restrictive protein diet. Her energy has returned, and her menses have been normal for the last two months. Her migraines disappeared," Dr. John Diamond affirms. "It merely meant that I needed to get the woman back to normal bowel function, off antibiotics, and onto probiotics all the time. Now she takes colon hydrotherapy on a regular once-a-month schedule. This patient will likely be forced to stay on her therapeutic program continuously."

BOARD-CERTIFIED GASTROINTESTINAL SURGEON LEONARD SMITH, MD, ENDORSES COLON HYDROTHERAPY

Thirty years ago, Leonard Smith, MD, of Gainesville, Florida, graduated from medical school and eventually became board-certified in general surgery by the American College of Surgery. For more than twenty-five years Dr. Smith has been in practice as a specialist in gastrointestinal surgery. He has dealt with all types of colon difficulties, including operations for overcoming colon cancer, colon diverticulitis, appendicitis, hemorrhoids, and numbers of other internal organ health problems. "I am very well acquainted with the colon's functions, and my true belief is that colon hydrotherapy is the perfect cleansing medium for preparing the patient for colonoscopy. It's a much better way of getting the human colon ready for an operation, than having a patient swallow a gallon of that usual pre-surgery solution known as 'Colon-Go-Litely.' Instead, colon hydrotherapy allows the patient to avoid this solution's noxious side effect of vomiting, diarrhea, abdominal cramping, and other troubles," Dr. Smith says. "Moreover, seriously ill patients tend to be chronically constipated, which results in generalized toxemia. It turns out that colon hydrotherapy is the gentlest and most effective treatment to take care of a sick person's constipation problem. My recommendation for cancer patients is that they should undergo frequent colon hydrotherapy procedures to make sure a colon's toxic burden is being kept at a minimum, while their bodies are trying to heal," affirms Dr. Smith. "Those cancer patients who take colon hydrotherapy often experience the elimination of their aches and pains, and have improved appetite and a higher tolerance of a tough healing process.

"I also believe that normally healthy people will find it valuable to take colon hydrotherapy every couple of months in order to experience how well one feels when the colon is truly empty. It's a fact that most people fail to fully evacuate the colon, something they don't realize. People undergoing colon hydrotherapy on a prevention basis become quite surprised at how much waste is removed by the procedure," Dr. Smith says.

"Without any reservation, I declare that my wish is to see it became an established procedure for many kinds of gastro-intestinal problems. If medical centers, hospitals, and clinics installed colon hydrotherapy departments, they would find such departments just as efficacious for patients as their present treatment areas which are devoted to physiotherapy," states Dr. Smith. "Such is my true belief, and I do endorse this therapeutic program."

GIVING COLON HYDROTHERAPY IS STANDARD PROCEDURE OF SHARDA SHARMA, MD

Located in Millburn, New Jersey, as a primary care physician for nearly twenty-six years, Sharda Sharma, MD, dispenses medical care of a multi-disciplinary nature to her patients. Dr. Sharma employs colon hydrotherapy, chelation therapy, massage therapy, acupuncture, Reiki manipulative therapy, and much more. She treats the body as a whole (holistically).

"I have trained and certified colon hydrotherapists working as part of my staff. Under my supervision, for the past year-and-a-half, they have been rendering care for constipation, abdominal cramps, allergies, and a variety of other conditions, including ten patients with hepatitis C. These hepatitis patients respond to colon hydrotherapy and do well," reports Dr. Sharma. "For instance, Mrs. Felicia, a forty-two-year-old high school teacher, had suffered with constipation — no bowel movements — for six days at a stretch. She was bloated, fatigued, lethargic, headachy, and crampy. My treatment choice for her was enzyme supplements and colon hydrotherapy twice weekly for thirteen weeks. These treatments solved the constipation problem for Mrs. Felicia. She goes to the toilet without having to sit there for long periods waiting, reading, meditating, or undergoing other mental or physical diversions."

MICHAEL GERBER, MD, USES COLON HYDROTHERAPY ROUTINELY

"I've had a colon hydrotherapy device in my office for twenty-five years," states Michael Gerber, MD, of Reno, Nevada. "My present staff person, who dispenses colon hydrotherapy under my jurisdiction, uses it for all types of patient difficulties. The basic concepts of the science have not changed much in the last twenty-five years; however, the colon hydrotherapy equipment has improved immensely. How the equipment works so effectively is nothing short of astounding. Registered with the FDA, current colon hydrotherapy equipment is safe. It contains temperature-controlled water mixing and back flow prevention valves, plus pressure and temperature sensors, and built-in chemical sanitizing units. Water purification units frequently are installed as well. Disposable single-use rectal tubes, and/or speculae are employed routinely for sterility."

Undergoing a session of colon hydrotherapy has you experiencing comfort and cleansing with no toxicity. Techniques utilized allow a small amount of water to flow into the colon, gently stimulating the colon's natural peristaltic action, to release softened waste. Dr. Gerber explains: "The inflow of a small amount of water and the release of waste may be repeated again and again. The removal of such waste encourages better colon function and elimination.

"During the treatment, most clothing can be worn. In addition, the patient is draped, or a gown is worn to ensure modesty. The patient's dignity is always maintained," Dr. Gerber affirms. "The benefits of colon hydrotherapy extend all the way from psychiatric improvement to constipation elimination."

CONDITIONS RESPONDING TO COLON HYDROTHERAPY CITED BY RHEUMATOLOGIST ARTHUR E. BRAWER, MD

"Colon hydrotherapy eliminates from the bowel the repository of accumulated waste material which may disadvantageously get absorbed. If this absorption takes place, it overwhelms the other purification organs such as the liver, the kidney, the skin, and the lungs. The toxin deposition which becomes lodged throughout the body's tissues and cells becomes capable of triggering a variety of illnesses," says rheumatologist Dr. Arthur E. Brawer. "There are lots of them."

Some disease indications that may respond well to colon hydrotherapy are:

Acne	Joint aches
Allergies	Memory lapses
Arthritis	Mouth sores
Asthma	Multiple sclerosis
Attention deficit disorder	Muscle pain
Body odor	Nausea
Brittle hair	Peptic ulcer
Brittle nails	Peripheral neuropathies
Chest pain	Pigmentation
Chronic fatigue	Poor posture
Cold hands & feet	Pot belly
Colitis	Seizures
Constipation	Skin rashes
Fibromyalgia	Spastic colon
Headaches	Toxic environmental exposure
Irritable bowel	Toxic occupational exposure

"COLON HYDROTHERAPY IS LIKE CLEANING BAKED LASAGNA FROM A PAN" SAYS PAMELA WHITNEY, ND

The late Dr. Whitney, education director of the New England Health Institute, was a naturopathic physician who practiced her profession in two locations: Braintree, Massachusetts, and Smithfield, Rhode Island. Here is how she described the physical action of colon hydrotherapy:

If ever you've baked lasagna and then attempted to sanitize the messy, leftover lasagna pan, you know the difficulty with getting it clean. For sponging such a food-caked pan it's usual for cooks to soak the pan overnight. Then they find that swabbing it the next day is easy.

Colon hydrotherapy accomplishes the same ease of cleansing on the inside of one's bowel. Using hydrotherapy, the colon's walls constantly get flushed with clear fluid, which serves to remove mucous plus some of their long-standing, caked-on fecal matter which contains hidden bacteria, parasites, Candida albicans-filled pockets, and other such pathological material.

Literature furnished by the International Association for Colon Hydrotherapy (I-ACT), located in San Antonio, Texas, defines colon hydrotherapy as a safe, effective method of removing waste from the large intestine, without the use of drugs. By introducing pure, filtered and temperature regulated water into the colon, the human waste is softened and loosened, resulting in evacuation through natural peristalsis. This flushing process usually is repeated a few times during a therapeutic session. Colon hydrotherapy is best used in combination with adequate nutrient and fluid intake, as well as with exercise. The modern and sophisticated technology applied today, manufactured through compliance with strict FDA guidelines, promotes both safety and sanitation of the procedure.

Dr. Pamela Whitney advised that her healing program for almost any condition frequently involved prescribing colon hydrotherapy. "I almost always refer my patients to undertake colon cleansing as the first part of my treatment. I do this for purposes of detoxification, since most people possess toxic bowels which may result in either constipation or diarrhea, both coming from the same sources of toxicity," she said. "The patient's toxins tend to kick back to their bloodstream and perpetuate numerous pathologies such as candidiasis, allergies, chronic fatigue, and other symptoms coming from a recalculation of accumulated physiological poisons.

"I use the services of at least three skilled colon hydrotherapists who practice near my two offices. I don't know of any patient receiving colon hydrotherapy who has not benefitted from it. Certainly the treatment will get a sluggish bowel refunctioning again. In my judgment, the action of just one colon hydrotherapy is an experience equivalent to someone undergoing twenty coffee enemas," said Dr. Whitney. "When we eat processed foods such as bread, pastas, sugars, and refined desserts, they hit the gastrointestinal tract like a glue-like substance and stick on the walls of one's GI tract. Thereafter, constipation with inflammation can develop, but colon hydrotherapy solves such a problem."

As is obvious, Dr. Pamela Whitney was a great advocate of colon hydrotherapy, which she prescribed as a standard part of her treatment.

CHRISTOPHER J. HUSSAR, DO, DDS, TOOK COLON HYDROTHERAPY

From his medical/surgical practice in Reno, Nevada, osteopathic physician and dental cavitation specialist Christopher J. Hussar, DO, DDS, offers the following personal statement. "I have enjoyed two colon hydrotherapy treatments when, at the time, I was experiencing partial bowel obstruction. Each colon hydrotherapy had me feeling better. It's my belief that this treatment should be recommended for any person who is having chronic constipation. Then, the local colon hydrotherapist can become a main factor in keeping that individual comfortable. I maintain that one should do whatever it takes to keep up with regular bowel movements. Colon hydrotherapy is a safe and natural laxative that works better than any other type.

"In Reno, I refer my patients who are in need of bowel cleansing to a colon hydrotherapist. The only reason that I don't refer people on a regular basis is because most of them arrive to see me from out of town. Therefore, I tell them to use the services of a skilled colon hydrotherapist located in their area, so that they can go for treatment often," says Dr. Hussar.

JANET BEATY, ND, TOOK TRAINING IN COLON HYDROTHERAPY

"My original training in colon hydrotherapy was when I administered it twenty-five years ago as part of my massage therapy program; that training went much deeper when I attended Bastyre University. I was one of several instructors in colon hydrotherapy at the naturopathic college," says Janet Beaty, ND, whose practice is in West Concord, Massachusetts. "Now I don't own the physical facilities for doing it in my office, but I regularly refer patients to a competent colon hydrotherapist nearby.

"My experience with the treatment is totally positive. I refer people to have it when they are constipated because their colons are not fully emptying, bringing on GI discomforts of some kind. My sense is that the patient must empty out old waste products so that there is no interference with healing modalities," states Dr. Beaty. "I am using colon hydrotherapy as my beginning treatment for detoxification, particularly for patients with congested bowels. While I focus on the gastro-intestinal aspects of colon hydrotherapy, I also prescribe it for the treatment of allergies, arthritis, and other health difficulties.

"If I had my druthers, I would get all of the patients with any health problems on colon hydrotherapy. Why I don't is because it entails the payment of cash-out-of-pocket and some people find the concept too 'kinky' even to imagine doing it," Dr. Beaty says. "Yet, probably most patients should receive at least one colon hydrotherapy during the course of taking care of themselves. It is a very helpful tool for nearly any patient in order to get the bowel peristalsis to work. An effective technique for stimulating such peristalsis is to start out with colon hydrotherapy using warm water, gradually decreasing the water temperature as treatment continues. This lower temperature tends to stimulate the bowel muscles. The cold temperatures cause good peristaltic action for retraining of the bowel.

"The ideal treatment program for the patient receiving colon hydrotherapy is from four to eight weeks. This time frame is necessary for unloading a bunch of toxins from the liver."

COLON HYDROTHERAPY USED BY JAMES P. CARTER, MD, DR PH

"After conducting a comprehensive digestive stool analysis on any patient suspected of having dysbiosis (poor intestinal hygiene), I attempt to wipe the bowel clean by prescribing colon hydrotherapy once a week, for three weeks. In my medical practice, I employ a registered nurse on staff to administer this treatment," says James P. Carter, MD, Dr PH, MS, of Mandeville, Louisiana. Dr. Carter is Professor and Head of the Nutrition Section at the Tulane University School of Medicine.

"Also I use colon hydrotherapy as part of an overall detoxification program, which may be combined with treatment from above such as drinking epsom salts, but both are not taken on the same day," he advises. "It promotes the second stage of liver detoxification, causing dissolved poisons to come out in the bile as a solvent.

"Colon hydrotherapy is an excellent detoxifier for the overindulgence of alcohol drinking and drug addictions of all kinds. Residues of drugs and other agents in the tissues are eliminated with colon hydrotherapy," says Dr. Carter. "It takes away any desire to use drugs or imbibe alcoholic beverages. Colon hydrotherapy should be part of nearly any addict's therapeutic regimen."

SEBASTIAN R. REYES, DOM, L.AC., DOCTOR OF ORIENTAL MEDICINE, LICENSED ACUPUNCTURIST IN PRACTICE OVER 40 YEARS

Benefits of Detoxification Through Colonics

Colon therapy is an ancient method of treatment and form

of detoxification. It never would have survived through the scientific era unless it had unquestionable value to its recipients.

It's a curious fact that medical practitioners seem to be either wholeheartedly in favor or vehemently against this procedure. Those who condemn it are nearly always those who have no knowledge of, or experience with, this therapy. Detoxification is the removal of the toxins from the body. You probably never considered the fact that your body, through improper diet, gets as dirty on the inside as it does on the outside!

Detoxification requires a special process for cleansing through specific diet, food supplements, juices, and other recommendations. Water can prevent such chronic diseases as cancer, cardiovascular problems, arthritis, diabetes, obesity, etc. Today's modern diet has excess animal proteins, fats, sugars, sodas, caffeine, and alcohol, which inhibit the functions of cells and tissues.

How Do You Know if You Are in Need of Detoxification?

When the body system is overwhelmed, its defense mechanism malfunctions. Symptoms may include fatigue, confusion, aggression, mental disorder, headaches, joint pain, respiratory problems, back pains, allergy, insomnia, mood changes, food allergies, etc.

My normal procedure to prepare a patient for a detoxification program is to check the blood pressure, and take urine and saliva samples. The urine and saliva samples reveal the patient's metabolism. This shows whether there are excessive carbohydrates, and whether alkaline or acidic conditions are present in the patient's system. With this information, we can design the proper diet program for the patient. The colonic administrator then determines how many sessions the patient needs.

The Three Elements of Natural Health: Mental, Spiritual, and Physical

When you begin to study natural health, it's important to start with the three elements that constitute good health: mental, spiritual, and physical harmony (balance). It all starts with knowledge of nutrition and the science of using specific nutritional techniques that have nothing to do with disease. A natural health doctor is a learned practitioner and teacher of sound nutrition. Also, this doctor has been trained in spiritual counseling techniques to be able to provide immeasurable spiritual and nutritional benefits to the patient. We do know that many terrible health problems simply disappear when a person concentrates on building their health instead of treating their disease. I believe that many "diseases" are not diseases at all but "conditions." A condition is something we have done to, or created in, our bodies, by what we eat and by our lifestyle.

Knowing the difference between diseases and conditions means that *we* have the responsibility for our health, since a condition is the result of nutritional deficiencies (wrong foods). These deficiencies, in turn, result in cellular contamination, and the body begins to deteriorate. Today people are dropping like flies from high blood pressure, blood sugar problems, strokes, kidney failure, tumors, arthritis, heart conditions, and more. In fact, the death rates from these problems (conditions) are at a higher level today than they were 20 years ago. Why? Because of inadequate nutrition! By knowing the patient's proper metabolism we can prescribe the proper diet, vitamins, minerals, and herbs, and how much of each is actually needed. The result can be perfect health.

The human body is a byproduct of the soil. The diet for a healthy individual should consist of many chemical elements, such as calcium, silicon, sodium, iodine, magnesium, potassium, zinc, and many others. These elements are found in fertile soil and transmitted to plant life where the chemicals of the soil become food for man. To enjoy perfect health, we must eat food containing the elements found in perfect fertile soil and be aware that quantity is not the same as quality. Heredity is no excuse. Many people think that good or bad health is the result of one's heredity. If this were true we could change the diet of some of those long-living foreigners to the diet of most Americans and they would continue to live practically disease-free.

Addictions and Low Blood Sugar

We hear about drug, alcohol, and cigarette addictions, but we almost never hear about sugar addiction. It is important to stay away from refined sugars, sweets, and carbohydrates. Our bodies need the proper kind of sugar. Without sugar in our blood we can go into a coma and die for lack of proper (oxygen) energy in the brain and other vital organs. Sugar (glucose) provides energy and thus is very important to our health. Low blood sugar symptoms—such as sudden headaches, uneasiness, sweats, lightheadedness, disorientation, and sudden loss of energy—are occurring more and more every day. Many people have been told to cope with this problem by snacking on something sweet. The problem is that when they do this the same problem reoccurs a few hours later and they have to repeat the whole process again.

People with low blood sugar may have a hard time keeping their weight down. Pregnant women have a difficult time carrying a baby for a full term, if they have a low blood sugar problem. There is a threat of a possible miscarriage when the sugar drops too low for a long period of time. In an extreme case of low blood sugar a coma can result and, ultimately, even death. This can happen any time, without much warning. I personally attribute many head-on automobile collisions, telephone pole collisions, and rear-enders on nothing more than low blood sugar with momentary blackouts happening while driving.

When Sugars Are Too High

When the sugar level goes up, the brain is deprived of oxygen and, like low blood sugar, this affects the ability to think. You can wake up in the morning tired and go to bed tired, irritable, impatient, with night urination, headaches, blurred vision, and dizziness. Your circulation becomes impaired, your hands and feet feel cold, and your legs "go to sleep" more frequently. Refined sugars are the culprits involved with both high and low blood sugar problems. Our bodies are created with a mechanism to properly metabolize the natural carbohydrates such as fruits, vegetables, and other natural foods. Refined sugars are absorbed so fast into the blood that it elevates the amount of fat in the bloodstream. This fat interferes with the function of natural insulin. If you have a strong pancreas, it will create enough insulin to overpower the fat and keep the blood sugar within tolerable levels, providing that the liver converts the sugar into fat faster than the pancreas can tolerate it. Along with the liver and the pancreas, the kidneys play a major part in excreting excess sugar from the blood and the body.

Watch Out for Artificial Sweeteners

It's important to maintain optimal health by improving your awareness about refined sugar and aspartame (marketed as NutraSweet, Equal, and Spoonful). Aspartame is a wood alcohol (methanol). The World Environmental Conference, in an article written by Nancy Markle (11/20/97), reported that there are over 5,000 products containing this chemical. The methanol toxicity mimics multiple sclerosis symptoms. There is absolutely no reason to take this product. *It is not a diet product, it makes your body crave more carbohydrates, and it will make you fat,* according to Dr. Roberts. If it says "sugar-free" on the label, *do not even think about eating or drinking it!* Senator Howard Metzenbaum passed a Senate bill that warned all pregnant women, mothers, and children of the dangers of aspartame. Learn the truth about aspartame—and then start by eliminating Diet Pepsi and Diet Coke. Reduce your intake of sweets (such as cookies, cakes, pies, bread and chocolates), and you may find that you will feel healthier and also lose inches and weight.

ROBERT D. IRONS, BS, COLUMBIA, MISSOURI

Robert D. Irons, BS, received his degree in biochemistry, and is currently working toward his Ph.D. in nutritional sciences. He began lecturing nationwide in 1998 at the age of 23, and has appeared at health conventions, on the radio, and on television promoting proper nutrition and cleansing. His lifelong experience with natural health has given him an age-old perspective on this subject.

A Unique Perspective

I believe I can offer a unique perspective to this subject of pooping. I, myself, have been doing it all my life. In fact, it was a focus in my household as I was growing up. You see, my father was deeply involved in promoting colon cleansing since the 1940s. It was such a common topic that we would often discuss it around the dinner table, to the extreme discomfort of our guests. After all, food and poop go "hand-in-hand." The quality and quantity of the first influences the quality and quantity of the second. This is a point that many people do not realize. Out of all the substances we take in from the environment, the one that has the most influence on our health is the food we eat. Furthermore, there are really only two main factors that contribute to our health: (1) the food and drink we consume, and (2) the genes which we inherited from our parents.

I'm quite proud that I have been endowed with the best of both. My father was Victor Earl Irons. Those of you who have been involved in nutrition and cleansing have probably heard of him. He had a long experience with foods, cleansing, and

151

the fight for health freedom. So, I have been endowed with good genes and proper knowledge about nutrition.

V. Earl Irons was born on January 23, 1895 (he was 80 years old when I was born!). Many changes to our food supply occurred during the 98 years he was alive. During his time he saw the introduction of refined white flour and sugar, pasteurized milk, margarine, microwaves, aluminum pots and pans, processed cheeses, and a host of other violations on our food supply. I cringe at the thought of him being alive today to see genetically modified organisms (GMO's) in our food supply, and the involvement of the USDA in setting the standards for organic food production. I know he would be outspoken against these ideas.

When my father was 40 years old (in 1935) his typical industrial diet led to his diagnosis of having an incurable disease: Marie Strumpell arthritis. His doctor told my father that within 20 years his spine would be bent so that he would not be able to raise his head any higher than his waist. The prognosis was that he would become a hunched-back old man, and there was nothing medical science could do to help.

My father had done some reading on health and nutrition. He said to his doctor, "I thank you for your time, Doctor, but I do not believe there is any such thing as an incurable disease." He adopted a regimen that was in complete harmony with what he deemed "natural law." This is a scientific principle that states:

> *In the mammal animal, every cell of the body is served by the blood, which nourishes the cell, replaces the "worn-out" parts, and carries away the waste products.*

My father reasoned that if his body was becoming diseased, he must change the quality of his blood so that it could properly nourish and detoxify the cells. His regimen was to eat only raw foods, and to do regular fasting and enemas. (This was in the 1930s, before colonics were widespread.) By doing this, he was supplying his bloodstream with perfect nutrition and perfect elimination.

The results were astounding. Within six months, he had no more pain in his back. After continuing this natural lifestyle for two years, he had x-rays taken of his spine. They showed a complete remission of all arthritic symptoms associated with his disease. Of course, his doctor had no logical explanation as to why his condition had disappeared. (This amazing recovery is not unique. We have seen thousands of people with chronic degenerative diseases such as cancer, heart disease, arthritis, etc. become completely healthy again. We only have to abide by nature's rules to achieve natural health.)

Such an event changes a man forever. He dedicated his life to teaching others about natural healing and preventative health maintenance. He co-founded the National Health Federation (NHF) as an organization that could lobby in Washington D.C. for protecting the individual's right to choose their medical — or nonmedical — treatment modality. Without these efforts, colonics, food supplements, and the alternative health care industry as a whole probably would have been controlled and/or disbanded by the U.S. government.

Did he live by a perfect diet for the rest of his life? No. I know of only one man who ever did: Dr. Norman Walker. But my father realized that the majority of food and drink he consumed should be truly nutrient-dense. This meant raw fruits and vegetables, good quality meats, and whole grains and flours — basically food that is unprocessed and not prepackaged. He also realized that his elimination should be complete and punctual. That is, he should have large, regular bowel movements (about 3) daily. If he ate 3 times a day, then he should defecate 3 times a day. Elimination should match intake. Whenever it did not, he would cleanse to make sure his elimination was perfect. Cleansing ensures that the bloodstream can effectively remove toxins from the cells. When the bloodstream and cells are healthy, the entire body will be healthy.

Through his lectures and teachings he helped George and Kay Shaffer. They had both been nurses and had both developed cancer. They adopted the 7-Day Cleansing Program advocated by my father as a way of life. However, instead of using an enema as suggested, George invented a home colonic board that could be used over his bathroom toilet. It allowed Kay and him to administer more effective colonic irrigation. When my father evaluated his creation, he declared that everyone should have access to one. In 1975, George and my father began producing the Colema Board (COLonic/enEMA) as the first home enema board kit. Time has proven that the use of the Colema Board dramatically improves the results one obtains during the 7-Day Cleansing Program. The matter people pass is truly astounding.

George and Kay lived cancer-free into their 80s. They, too, shared their gift of knowledge with others. When people contacted my father requesting guidance on the cleansing program, he sent them to George and Kay Shaffer. People came from all over the world for cleansing. Their most notable and influential guest was Dr. Bernard Jensen. Dr. Jensen came to the Shaffers with his own health problems, for he knew nothing of colon cleansing at the time. The Shaffers taught him all they knew, and Dr. Jensen went on to write the book, *Tissue Cleansing Through Bowel Management*. This important work has been a powerful tool for introducing people to fasting and cleansing.

My father's approach to life served him well. He started his second family at the age of 72, and fathered his last child (me) at the age of 80. He died at the age of 98 with *no signs or symptoms of disease*. His family carries on his teachings and his work through the companies Mr. Irons founded: V.E. Irons, Inc., Sonne's Organic Foods, and Springreen Products.

You had your first colonic when you were HOW OLD?

I see it as a blessing that I grew up in the environment he provided. I have been able to teach my wife and family the importance of proper nutrition and cleansing. But looking back, I see my childhood as, shall we say, unique. For instance, I remember when I was 7 years old I wanted to play hooky from school. "If you are sick enough to stay home from school, then you better take a colonic," was his response. So, I went to our dedicated colonic bathroom to take a treatment so that I could stay home from school. In fact, any time I had the sniffles, a cough, or any sign of a cold, I was directed to "go and take a colonic." It was nothing strange to me, just like brushing my teeth. Later, I realized that not everyone did this type of thing. But now I realize that these mild symptoms are the first signs of a compromised immune system. The act of taking a colonic flushes immunogenic (toxic) substances from the colon and the bloodstream (indirectly). Come to think of it, I never had a cold growing up until I began eating the school's cafeteria food.

Did you talk about this at school?

Imagine what it was like for me at a public school. I learned quickly not to discuss this topic with my peers or my teachers. In the third grade, I kept my mouth shut while our teacher demanded that the hooligan responsible for putting his dirty shoes on the boy's toilet seat step forward. I didn't know any better. I had squatted on the toilet my entire life. From that experience, I learned to lift the seat, stand on the bowl, and wipe it off afterwards. It was my potty training, so to speak.

What do you mean, you squat?

Every mammal in the natural world squats to defecate. I am only doing things instinctually. As I grew up, I tried to confide in some of my closest friends. I knew that all my friends were clueless to the principles of health that I was taught. But, I thought that I should offer some suggestions now and again. One time in particular I tried to relate to my friend, Ray, about the proper position to have a bowel movement. I told him that when he *sits* on a toilet seat, this unnatural position causes a kink to form in the colon. The feces can't move efficiently through this kink, so some of it gets left inside the colon after a bowel movement. [This book has enlightened us to the idea that material left inside the colon can harbor the growth of putrefactive bacteria and parasites, and contribute to constipation.] I told him how it was natural for animals to squat; when humans are out in the woods we have to squat; and before the advent of the toilet every man, woman, and child squatted. It took some time, but I convinced him that constipation was part of the problem behind his severe acne. A real feat, considering he didn't think diet had anything to do with anything. When he told me he tried it, he said he started cracking up because he felt like a monkey. I had never thought of it that way. Nevertheless, Ray didn't put much credence in my words, so his problems persisted.

I find that it is difficult for younger people who have their health to really care about their nutrition. In our youth, our life energy is high and our bodies can still take much abuse before it shows. We feel that we are invincible and we will never get old and decrepit. In reality, the abuses we inflict on our bodies have a cumulative effect. The harder we are on our bodies when we are young, the more damage will show up as we get older. If our lifestyle and eating habits do not change, our bodies will not be able to cope with abuse, and our health may fail completely — becoming riddled with chronic diseases. When this happens, we will do everything we can—and spend any amount of money—to get our health back.

Waste not, want not. The earlier we start eating mainly natural, unprocessed food and cleansing regularly, the better health we will have into our twilight years. The objective is to add life to our years, and not just years to our life. Would you rather age gracefully and die in peace, or cling to those last few years of life in a comatose state with machines and drugs as the only means for survival? The choice is yours, and the sooner you make the right choice, the better your life will become.

Orthodox medicine is very expensive. Our present health care system cannot afford geriatric care for every individual. It is clear to those who know the system that within a few short years there will not be enough health care funds to pay for the growing elderly population. When we reach an age of need, there may not be any money left to treat our diseases. Doctor visits, hospitalization, drugs, blood tests, electromagnetic scans, biopsies, etc., are involved in the orthodox treatment of disease and are very costly in terms of money, time, and overall health.

The natural road to health is far more inexpensive and effective because it focuses on *prevention* instead of the *treatment* of disease after it is established. "An ounce of prevention is worth a pound of cure." The costs of natural remedies are trivial compared to the cost of orthodox medicine. Fasting and limiting your food intake is a very good way to cut down on your food bill and enhance your longevity. Prevention of disease using natural remedies requires increasing the nutrient and enzyme density of your dietary intake, and cleansing to give your body every possible means for evacuating detrimental biochemicals. However, this preventative approach to medicine takes more discipline than simply popping a pill or having surgery. It is long-term care, rather than a short-term fix.

To put this in the context of this book: Natural health care would address bowel problems with continuous fasting and colonics until the problems subside and health is regained, whereas orthodox medicine would suppress the symptoms of the bowel problem with drugs until a disease state results, and a portion of the bowel needs to be removed by colostomy. In this situation, health is never regained. Instead, a compromise occurs in which you are able to continue your poor eating habits, but you lose natural bowel function and have to defecate into a bag. This is not the way.

Has anybody really looked at their success rate?

How successful is orthodox medicine at treating our degenerative diseases? While no direct studies have looked at the efficacy of orthodox medical treatment, we can look at the general health status of the population. The U.S. Government for Health Statistics stated in 1994 that 85% of adult Americans are afflicted with "chronic diseases" (such as allergies, recurring headaches, fatigue, heart disease, cancer, etc.). Their definition of a chronic disease is one that *cannot be cured with medical intervention.* So, the great majority of Americans are living with some sort of disease. Are we really producing any cures with the billions of dollars that we spend on medical treatments, drug development, and research? To those with open minds and eyes, it is obvious that we are looking in the wrong direction. By examining disease and death, instead of health and life, we have locked ourselves into a concentric circle of confusion. We will never truly understand health when all we study is disease.

The natural methods of healing that I propose are in complete harmony with nature, and are derived from the study of life. Over a hundred years ago scientists discovered that perfect health could exist if an organism is given (1) *perfect nutrition* and (2) *perfect elimination* of its metabolic byproducts. In addition, we also know for a fact that if we reduce the dietary intake of an organism by 30%, the life span of that organism dramatically increases. The principles of nutrition, fasting, and cleansing achieve nature's requirements for vibrant life.

The future of health care from a biochemist's perspective

This book has taken the reader through so many different emotions, I feel I must bring up another: fear. I am deeply afraid of what the future holds with the advent of genetic engineering. The pharmaceutical, biotechnology, agrochemical, and medical industries are becoming one large conglomerate owned by very few companies. This alliance brings the pharmaceutical world into agriculture. They are using their position of power to manipulate our food supply so that immunizations and medications can be administered very cheaply and with control. Bananas and potatoes will soon carry inoculations, insulin, or a variety of other "designer drugs." No more shots or pills. This is a new dawn in easy-to-administer medication. Hippocrates' famous statement, "Let medicine by thy food, and food thy medicine," will take on a new, sinister meaning.

What has it taken for us to come to this point? Are humans so prone to genetic degeneration that we must resort to modifying our food supply and genetic makeup to survive? No. The truth is that our food supply has become so far removed from its natural state that it has lost most of the health-promoting qualities it once possessed. The result is long-term, subtle malnutrition which finally manifests itself as cumulative degeneration in the form of allergies, arthritis, cancer, diabetes, heart disease, osteoporosis ... the list goes on and on.

Nature has its own view of genetics. This view has been established over thousands of years. The protein, carbohydrate, fat, vitamins, and minerals that we consume dictate our genetic potential. Science has just realized in the last 15 years that the food we eat interacts with our DNA to elicit "nutrient regulation of gene expression." Why, then, do they not look to natural foods for the answer? Well, I guess they are looking to foods, in a way. But, now we are trying to master and change it, rather than learn from it. We must not let our entire food supply become engineered to suit the "needs" of the masses. We must be able to retain our freedom of choice to eat organic foods that are not tainted or changed in any way by man.

So, I am fearful of what the future holds, and in what kind

of world my children will live. V. Earl Irons would be fearful, too. But he would be fighting it tooth and nail. I know he would oppose the USDA's involvement with the certification of organic standards for the U.S. This is not the way. We can still live in harmony with nature. All we have to do is demand it.

If I can offer any closing words of advice to you, it is this. Drink predominantly water—not sodas, coffee, or alcohol. Eat predominantly raw, whole foods from good sources (farmer's markets, coops, or grown yourself). Don't worry about every little morsel of food you put into your mouth. Indulge a little, and enjoy life. Just make sure you cleanse to make amends for those subtle pleasures.

DAVID RAMSEY, DC, CAMPBELL, CALIFORNIA

There I was, lying on an exam table in the hospital emergency room, in severe pain, as the emergency room doctor was frantically trying to dislodge a bowel blockage that was, as he described, "as big as a large grapefruit."

The two months leading up to this traumatic night were the most miserable of my life. They were filled with miserable days, rectal bleeding from hemorrhoids and fissures, and sleepless nights from all the pain and from having to get up to take aspirin every few hours. As a doctor of chiropractic I don't advocate taking drugs, but I was in a desperate situation.

As I was contemplating whether I would need hemorrhoid surgery or a surgical procedure of a sphincterotomy (which had been recommended to me by a proctologist several years earlier) I called my brother-in-law, a surgeon, for advice. When I asked him what it was like to go through this procedure, he began to tell me about an old cowboy he had performed the surgery on. The patient described his first bowel movement following his surgery as "trying to pass the sun with barbed wire wrapped around it."

Well, thank God I never had to have the surgery. The emergency room doctor was successful in removing the blockage from my bowel. When my bowels started working again I started to heal, and the pain subsided in the next few weeks.

About a week before the emergency room visit I called my old friend, Loree Jordan, and she got me in for a colonic, which helped a little. But I had let this problem go on too long, and the blockage was too severe. In retrospect, I should have gone to Loree for a series of colonics before this problem turned into a nightmare. I just put it off.

Loree also asked me if I had been taking the "bowel blaster" program she had gotten me on so many years before. I had to admit to her that I hadn't, even though over the years I had suffered from chronic constipation. When I first started taking her recommended program years ago, everything she said would happen actually did, and more. I must admit I felt great. But alas, I didn't stay in the habit. Thus, the years of colon neglect took their toll and, well, you heard where it got me: in the emergency room!

Now a day does not pass without my taking the bowel blaster program, and I feel better than I've felt in years. I've also incorporated Loree's colon health philosophy into my practice and have observed that toxic bowel syndrome, or *dysbiosis*, is the root cause of a myriad of health problems in our society. I routinely tell my patients that almost all health problems can be traced to problems in either the nervous system or digestive system.

Once I started incorporating into my practice diagnostic procedures and treatments centering on the digestive system, I really started to see some interesting patterns emerge in my patients. It was amazing to me how many people report having bowel movements once a day, or even as infrequently as every other day or less. It seems to be the general consensus of my patients that, if they have a bowel movement once a day or less, it is considered normal.

I am seeing more and more how unusual it is to find a person who has 2 to 3 healthy bowel movements per day. Another common observation is that patients with the most challenging health symptoms such as chronic fatigue, immune system disorders, fibromyalgia, allergies, etc., all have 100% correlation with dysbiosis, or toxic bowel syndrome.

We need to stop abusing our digestive systems with fast foods and toxins. We need to start drinking more water and consuming more fiber and healthy organic foods, so that our gastrointestinal systems are clean and functional. At all costs we want to guard against autointoxication setting the stage for a disease process. Parasitic infestation, colon cancer, and intestinal disorders are running rampant in our society. Loree has once again stepped up to the plate to educate the public about the importance of detoxification and our health. Anyone struggling with health challenges, or anyone choosing to maintain their health, must take this book to heart.

If more people had access to this information, the number of cases of colon cancer alone would decrease dramatically. Not only cancer but colitis, parasites, candidiasis (yeast syndrome), immune system suppression, skin problems, some cases of low back pain, bloating, chronic fatigue, and fibromyalgia would be reduced—the list goes on and on.

I am very grateful for all that Loree has taught me, for I feel that she has literally saved my life. This vital information could save the lives of countless other people.

I work with three primary tenets of naturopathy, adapted from Jim Sharp's book, Basic Principles of Total Health: Harmonious Integration of Body, Mind and Spirit:

1. *The primary cause of disease is the accumulation of unnecessary wastes which are not properly eliminated, resulting in poison retention and subsequent disease.*

2. *Your body is designed to support optimal function. Listen to its signals.*

3. *Given the proper environment, your body has the power to heal itself and return to its normal healthy state.*

– Elson Haas, MD, *The Detox Diet*

CHAPTER 13

■ ■ ■ ■ ■ ■ ■ ■ ■ ■ ■

Children, Nutrition, and Potty Talk

Parents want to do right by their children, but when it comes to nutrition, what's "right" isn't always apparent. Good nutrition for our children involves more than providing regular meals and keeping the junk food out of the cabinets.

PARENTS AS ROLE MODELS

As parents we have the ultimate responsibility to impart knowledge about health and to model healthful behaviors to our children. Our behaviors have an impact on our children, either negative or positive. We know that children practice and imitate our behavior, whether it is our eating habits or our communication style. Children see and follow the main models they have: their parents' examples.

Probably like you, I did not question or negotiate food choices while growing up in my parents' home. I never went to bed hungry; as far as I knew I was eating well. Knowledge I've gained since then has led me to believe otherwise.

I grew up in my family, eating foods that I would not even consider at this point in my life. It was cereal and milk for breakfast. Typical school lunches were peanut butter and jelly or bologna and cheese sandwiches, potato chips, some sweets (cupcakes or cookies), and fruit. My favorite snack after school was marshmallow creme spread (from a jar) between two graham crackers.

My mom was Italian. I remember going to my great-grand-mother's house to watch her make homemade raviolis with a special rolling pin. They were so delicious. We ate a lot of pasta, garlic bread, salami, and cheese. That was the Italian way.

We also ate a lot of meat at the dinner table. My grand-father was part owner of a ranch and we had access to lots of beef. Our freezer in the garage was always stocked full of beef. My dad, Bob, was the "King of the Barbecue." He barbecued everything. My parents built a house in the country when I was 8 years old; my dad had a special indoor barbecue pit built into the kitchen. The man was committed to barbecuing. Growing up with my dad's barbecuing talents turned me into a connoisseur of barbecued steak and barbecued chicken—if it was barbecued I loved it. Believe me, I got my fill. I amazed my dad by eating a huge plate of steak and then hovering over his plate and asking him if I could finish his. He was under-standably surprised when, in my 30s, I became a strict vegetarian for eight years.

WE DON'T TALK ABOUT "THAT" IN OUR FAMILY

I don't know how things were in your household, but we did not talk about nutrition or bowel movements in our home. I remember getting the sex education talk and the menstruation talk, but nothing about bowel movements. Was I constipated? Did I poop regularly? What was regular? No questions asked. Nothing ... nada. It wasn't that my parents didn't care. They probably didn't realize the importance of discussing pooping habits with their kids. It was never suggested that I be given an enema when I was sick (as I am going to suggest to parents reading this book). It just wasn't talked about!

I remember when I was about 12 years old my mom went

to a chiropractor's office for colonic treatment. She never openly discussed it in our family; I just have a vague memory of her going to these colonic appointments. The only thing I remember her saying to me was that her stomach was flat after she got a treatment. Since my mom passed away when I was 18 years old, I was not given the opportunity to learn from her the benefits of these colonics. I did not know what a colonic was, or what its real purpose was.* Then, 18 years after her death, I become a certified colon hydrotherapist ... What is that universal message?

CHILDREN AND NUTRITION

All the food recommendations—food combining and nutrition principles—apply to children as well. Children can get their foundation in life with lots of nature's pure foods. This is the time to instill in our children good eating and eliminating habits. They go hand in hand. Good diets, with lots of fruits and vegetables, will provide good elimination. A diet of processed junk foods will encourage constipation and a sluggish intestinal system in children.

Children need to learn what foods produce what results in their bodies. For example, if your child wants to eat only cheese sandwiches with white bread, or only macaroni and cheese, think of how it will affect the intestinal system. These foods are hard to eliminate because they create paste or glue in the intestinal system. This is a diet that predisposes children to constipation. Children need to be taught that fruits and vegetables are natural foods, and that they need lots of them in their diet to stay healthy. When pregnant, most women watch their own diet fastidiously, and will take many vitamins for their baby's

---

* My mom was tuned into colonics, an important component of vital health, but as this book shows, it is a combination of factors that keeps a person free from cancer. She may have been genetically predisposed, but I will never know.

health. That is only the first phase of motherhood. The next phase is feeding your growing children nutrient-rich foods that support their growth, foster their learning capabilities, and send them into adulthood with a healthy body.

I did not start learning about proper nutrition until my sons were about 6 and 8 years old. Our dietary makeover was not without its challenges. They already had many years of bad nutrition habits behind them. They'd love to tell you how I tortured them with carrot juice, coconut milk (which I made myself), and healthy snacks. They say they were always embarrassed because their friends would come over and there was "nothing good to eat," which meant: no Doritos, ice cream, cookies, etc. Since I could not expect them to be perfect, I came up with a plan. We would have "Bojangles Day" in our house. On Bojangles Day my sons would be allowed as much junk food as they wanted within a 24-hour period. What was left over (at the 24-hour mark) was thrown out. What was interesting about this family ritual was that the boys noticed they did not feel well after eating junk foods. They noticed stuffy noses from drinking milk and lack of energy from eating all the sugar. I wasn't thrilled that they wanted to scarf all this junk food, but it was a win-win situation and it kept my sons from feeling completely deprived. The other 90 to 95% of the time their diets were pretty clean. Expecting absolutely perfect behavior from children is a set-up for failure and resentment.

My older son, Brandon, shared a story with me about being embarrassed about our health foods in the cupboard, and getting teased when his friends came over. Brandon and his friend Jeremy were rummaging through the cabinets one night (he was about 14 at the time) and found a bottle of a liquid concentrate called Herbal Punch. Brandon and Jeremy just howled with laughter at the thought of making herbal punch. I mean, they wanted the hard stuff: Coke, root beer, Pepsi— anything but herbal punch!

Just a few months ago we had the pleasure of having Jeremy and a few of his friends over to our new house. As a joke, Brandon (now in his early 20s) and I decided we would bring out the Herbal Punch and offer it to Jeremy. The look on his face was priceless. We were all hysterical with laughter. It was a very Kodak moment.

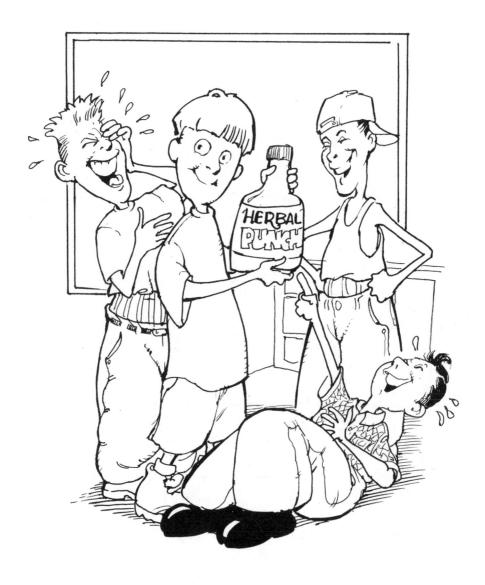

Hold That Ice Cream!

Ice cream manufacturers aren't required to list additives used in their products. These Arizona health organization findings may scare you right out of the grocery store. Here's what was found, even in the "quality supermarket and specialty brand ice cream."

Lice-killing chemical peperona. Used as a vanilla flavoring.

Rubber cement ingredient butyraldehyde. This not only makes great glue, but gives ice cream a nut-like flavor.

Paint remover and antifreeze chemical diethyl glucol. A cheaper emulsifier than egg.

Nitrate solvent benzyl acetate. Ice cream manufacturers think it's a great strawberry flavoring.

The chemical aldehyde C-17 used in rubber and plastics, and in exotic flavors of ice cream. Danger: flammable!

Leather and textile cleaner ethyl acetate. Dry cleaners know about its harmful vapors, but do our bodies have to find out the hard way? Used in various ice cream flavors.

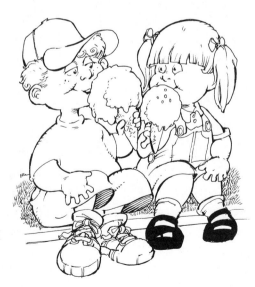

Natural ice cream from the health food store contains no chemical additives or flavorings, and as an extra bonus it's free of refined sugar. So next time your kids ask for ice cream, pass the regular grocery store and head for the health food store.

POTTY TALK

◆ Don't be embarrassed to talk openly with your children about bowel habits. It is vital to their health.

◆ Be informed. Do not buy into advice from the family doctor or pediatrician not to worry if your child's bowels only move 3 or 4 times a week or less.

◆ Help your children make good food choices; lots of fruits and vegetables to keep their bowels working properly.

◆ Help your children understand that the call to poop or eliminate is important. They should stop what they are doing to go to the bathroom. Don't let a child get in the habit of holding a bowel movement to get to it later.

◆ Encourage your children to be patient and not try to hurry up while sitting on the toilet. Let them take adequate time to allow the entire stool to be passed.

◆ Encourage your children to get adequate physical activity and not become sedentary, sitting in front of the TV, computer, or stereo. Physical activity encourages a healthy bowel.

◆ Instruct your children on the importance of washing their hands thoroughly after using the bathroom. The risk of infection of e-coli and parasites is real and must be taken seriously. (Chapter 14 about parasites addresses some issues of safety for children around pets.)

In *Colon Health for Children: A Parent's Guide,* Catherine Cavanaugh, RN, states:

> *From my observations, the bowel habits of children today appear to be worse than at any time in the 20 years of my nursing career. Discussions with nurses whose experience predates my own reinforce this conclusion, and several recent pediatric health care books mention this very same fact. In one excellent text Dr. Jack Schiller mentions that he frequently encounters parents who assure*

him that their child has regular daily bowel movements, but nevertheless he finds the child to be constipated (Schiller, 1982). He attributes this to the fact that even though a movement may be taking place every day, only part of the day's accumulation of waste is being passed, and the remainder gradually builds up and clogs the colon.

Ms. Cavanaugh goes on to say that, in reviewing her records for the past 13 years, she found that she was called upon to remove nearly twice as much fecal-impacted material in children and teens in the last 5 years than in the previous 10 years combined. The reasons for this appear to be worsening dietary habits, lack of sufficient exercise, and inadequate parental supervision of bowel function (often a result of poor advice from uninformed pediatricians and family medical doctors). Her experience as a nurse for more than a decade has shown Ms. Cavanaugh that this lack of emphasis by parents in ensuring that their children develop regular bowel habits is a major contributor to the overall poor physical condition of kids today.

Physician uses colon hydrotherapy for constipated eight-year-old

"One of my more significant cases was Tommy, an eight-year-old boy with the most awful constipation anyone could imagine," says former general surgeon and emergency medicine specialist Paul Flashner, MD of Wellesley, Massachusetts. Observing their superior results for his patients, Dr. Flashner has more recently adapted his treatment techniques almost completely to complementary and alternative medicine (CAM). Most definitely, he has incorporated colon hydrotherapy as a regular CAM technique.

"Tommy's constipation was really bad. He wouldn't have a bowel movement for a week at a time. Recognizing the dangers of physiological toxicity, his parents took their son for consultation with numerous gastroenterologists. The child had been subjected to colonoscopy a dozen times, but nothing could be found as the source of his blockage. Laxatives hardly helped at all. There was no diagnosis except that he suffered severely from constipation," confirms Dr. Flashner. "Then the parents found their way to me so that the boy might undergo examination and treatment one more time. They described their eight-year-old's condition.

"I improved the child's diet and removed all junk foods. Then I instigated an exercise program, had him drink lots of water, balanced his colonic flora, and added fiber supplements. But most vital for Tommy's welfare is that he took colon hydrotherapy under my prescription. The beneficial effect was dramatic, for within six months he was experiencing a natural and normal bowel movement every day. No laxatives were involved in his progress," stated Dr. Flashner. "Now the child does not need to consult me anymore; still, he continues his colonic cleansing four times a year. It's been two years that Tommy remains in excellent physical condition."

With regard to the relationship of the colon to the rest of the body's organs, Dr. Norman Walker states: "Beginning in childhood and through adolescence, discipline (or lack of it), is greatly responsible for this condition (of poor bowel health)."

WHEN CHILDREN ARE SICK

I am going to reiterate that the principles of healing children and adults are the same. The body must be allowed to do its healing work. The advantage children have over adults is that they heal quickly and, hopefully, they do not have years of improper nutrition, drugs, and other toxins in their systems. I need to emphasize the importance of opening up the bowel by way of enemas or home colonic treatments when children are sick. When the bowel is cleared the child's body is able to deal with the infection or virus by way of *all* the eliminative channels. Until the colon is cleaned out, there is no place for the other toxins to move. It used to be common practice for Grandma to give her family members enemas when someone was sick. Unfortunately we have gotten away from Grandma's basics and have turned into a "pill for every ill" society.

Let me share with you this story from Dr. Bernard Jensen. Even though it refers to a young man, not a child or infant, the principle is the same. Dr. Jensen and Dr. Glenn J. Sipes went on an emergency call. On arriving, they found a young man about 26 years of age, red as a beet and oozing liquid from his skin. He had extreme pain throughout his entire body and a very high fever. Dr. Sipes tapped the man's bowel with his fingers and asked when he'd had his last bowel movement. The young man said he couldn't remember. Dr. Sipes turned to the mother and asked her to prepare an enema, as the young man needed one right away. She asked what an enema was. There wasn't a thing in that house to give an enema with, but Dr. Sipes was a man who could always find his way out. He went outside and down to the creek, and cut a piece of reed about 2½ feet long. He had the man's mother fill up a kettle with warm water. He cleaned the pith out of the reed with baling wire, then took some of the warm water and blew it into the rectum, causing the man to eliminate. This procedure was repeated for over an hour. In an hour and a half, the man's fever had dropped to normal. There was no more redness of the skin and no more pain in his body.

This example is pretty straightforward and solidly illustrates my point. This is only one of the many stories that confirm the importance of opening up the bowel and allowing the healing process to occur.

CAN CHILDREN HAVE COLONIC TREATMENTS?

Absolutely! Children whose parents start them out with a regular bowel cleansing education at an early age are more likely to stay with the program through life than those who are introduced to the program in teen years or later. The age at which children should begin receiving colonic treatment varies. Usually 5 to 8 years old is the preferred starting age. Parents can begin the routine of regular bowel cleansing using enemas or the Colema Board (home colonic unit) for their children. This way children grow up feeling comfortable with occasional bowel cleansing as part of their normal routine. Colonic irrigation can assist in the following areas of children's health care:

◆ For the purpose of developing good health habits and a preventive maintenance program at an early age. Ideally, the child will be introduced to colon care while still in good health and before any bowel problems have had a chance to develop.

◆ For the relief of temporary or occasional constipation, when no more than a single routine cleansing enema would be required.

◆ To assist in the correction of habitual, long-term constipation and bowel retraining.

STAY AWAY FROM THE DRUGSTORE

The other point I want to emphasize is that running to the pharmacy and loading up on drugs for your child is just a temporary solution to the problem. This is a no-win situation because drugs will just drive the illness back into the tissues of the body, to be dealt with later. I will talk about these healing principles at length in Chapter 19, which discusses the Hering's Law of Cure. Instead of turning to drugs, arm yourself with knowledge and learn a more natural way to assist your child in getting well.

Once I learned these principles I practiced them with my family. I have to say that from the time my sons were 6 and 8 (after Brandon's ear problem was resolved), they were rarely sick. On occasion, when they did become sick, they took herbs and supplements and also spent time on the Colema Board (home colonic unit). When I wrote for the local newspaper in Hollister, California, I wrote many articles on how to use herbs instead of drugs to treat childhood illnesses. I consulted with many parents and taught them how to manage illness without resorting to drugs. When parents changed their children's diet and supported the immune system, going to the pediatrician became unnecessary.

When I saw mothers running their children to the doctor every other week for every cough and cold that came around, I was grateful for the knowledge that I had. Even though my sons (now young men) have active and busy lives and don't always follow natural nutrition, I feel that they have these principles in their consciousness. When they do have the misfortune of becoming sick they go directly to natural herbal remedies and know how to assist their bodies in the healing process.

Supporting your children means becoming an activist: making a conscious effort to acquire knowledge (i.e., reading books like this), shopping carefully, becoming a label sleuth so you know what you are feeding your family, and loving and supporting your children when their best efforts to make good food choices are challenged by peer pressure. Also, support can come from well-planned meals to avoid reliance on fast foods in these hectic times.

Trying to keep it all together as a parent can be an over-whelming challenge. I always say, "Progress, not perfection."

I would like to share a story I wrote when my sons were in grade school. I think every parent can relate to this lighter side of raising kids.

"What's For Dinner, Mom?"

Whatever happened to the good old-fashioned meal? With hectic lifestyles, it seems that moms, dads, and kids are all going in different directions. Mealtimes are not what they used to be.

Somewhere between the alarm going off in the morning and getting out the door, mealtimes become a fast-paced insanity game of Beat the Clock. In my family we all move at different speeds. Trying to get everyone at the breakfast table at the same time is frustrating at best. With a glimpse of the last backpack going out the door, I assess the damages. With half-eaten toast, jam stuck on the outside of jars, drawers all hanging open, I am wondering if Hurricane Hugo just passed through my kitchen. My kids pack their lunches for school, but you have to watch kids. They will of course pack 40 granola bars, 20 bags of raisins, and no veggies or fruit. If I shop on the weekend and buy enough lunch goodies to last all week, by Tuesday everyone is complaining that *there is nothing good for lunch!* That is because they have inhaled everything in sight and all that is left is brown bananas!

Do they care that I paid $39.95 per box for 12 granola bars at the health food store? Do they care that I go nuts because I see money evaporate in the grocery store? Remember when $100 would buy 2 weeks' worth of food? Now if I'd buy $100 worth, the grocery clerk would probably ask, "Is this a takeout order or do you want to eat it here?" My husband doesn't think it is very funny that I just spent $100 at the grocery store and still don't have anything to fix for dinner.

Children turn into locusts after 3 p.m. when they return home from school. Anything not nailed down is munching material, meant to be inhaled. Even though I've stocked the shelves and refrigerator for another 3 p.m. locust attack, with plenty of fruit, celery, carrots, and such, my kids still insist, "Mom, there's nothing good to eat."

By the time I get home, I notice Hurricane Hugo has once again whipped through my kitchen. I stumble over sweatshirts, backpacks, and lunch boxes as I tread my way to my so-called private sanctum to peel off my pantyhose. I am no architect, but mentally I am already designing the ideal family kitchen and dining room. It will have completely tiled walls and a cement floor with a drain in the center. That way I could just hose it all down after meals. I no sooner get my pantyhose peeled off than the bedroom door bursts open and those gifts from God begin the seemingly religious chant: "What's for dinner, Mom?"

I find myself in a trance, staring at the sacred refrigerator, whose whirring motor seems to have a stronger heartbeat than mine, as I survey its remaining contents: wilted broccoli and a half bottle of Gulden's mustard. Now, the key word in my state of mind is "fast." Even though, by profession, I am a holistic health expert who preaches the value of quality, non-junk food for kids, I am totally brain dead at this point. My kids begin another Gregorian-like religious chant that they learned around the age of 6: "Pizza, pizza, *pizza!*" I slowly dial the number of their favorite pizza parlor, and ask, "How fast can you deliver?"

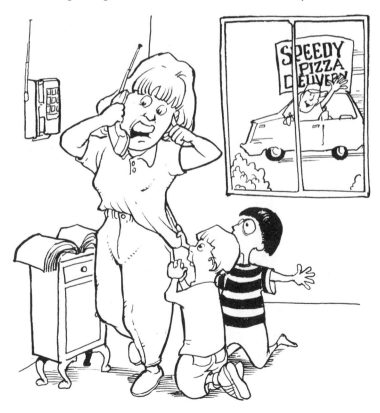

HANG IN THERE

You know that a hectic lifestyle can sometimes get the best of us, but the more open we are with our children, the more we teach the value of good health, good elimination, and good hygiene, the better our opportunity to raise healthy adults. It all starts with you as conscious parents. Good luck!

The Resource Guide (Chapter 24) lists some excellent books that discuss nutrition and natural remedies for childhood ailments in more detail. Please consult your health food store for other books on health programs for children. Even though we have not discussed vaccinations for children in this chapter, the Resource Guide also includes some reference material on this very important subject. If you have children you will find this vital information helpful.

CHAPTER 14

■ ■ ■ ■ ■ ■ ■ ■ ■ ■ ■

Parasites and Worms (and Other Creepy-Crawly Critters)

Make no mistake about it, worms are the most toxic agents in the human body. They are one of the primary underlying causes of disease and the most basic cause of a compromised immune system.

– Hazel Parcell, DC, ND, Ph.D.

DID YOU SAY PARASITES AND WORMS?

This chapter will be a bitter pill to swallow and by far the most shocking. Just the idea of parasites and worms crawling around in your body is enough to send you into shock and denial. All I can say is, take a deep breath, keep an open mind, and review the facts. Now, to add insult to injury, as your body is working overtime to handle, digest, and clean up your own wastes, worms and parasites find a perfect breeding ground between the thick mucus coating and your colon wall. And as they eat our food, their excrement becomes a source of toxic poisoning which goes right into the bloodstream and overloads the liver. Yes, you heard me right. As if black, goopy snakes coming out of the colon are not grotesque enough, now you can add worms and parasites to the list.

With the filth and toxins we have created in our bodies, we have provided a perfect environment for the invasion of

- ◆ Parasites outrank cancer as man's deadliest enemy on a worldwide basis.

- ◆ It is believed that 90% of the population is infested with worms.

- ◆ Over 100,000 Americans die annually due to these diseases.

parasitic scavengers. I always say that maggots cannot live in a clean garbage can. Parasites cannot live in a clean, healthy body.

I learned an awful lot about parasites from Ann Louise Gittleman's classic, *Guess What Came to Dinner*. In her book, which was first published in 1993 and updated in 2001, I discovered that the word "parasite" is from the Greek word *para* (meaning beside) and *sitos* (meaning food). A parasite is described as an organism that derives its food, nutrition, and shelter by living in or on another organism. A parasite lives off the host—you and me. Americans today are host to more than 130 different kinds of parasites, ranging from microscopic organisms to foot-long tapeworms. Parasites know no socio-economic or geographic boundaries. Practically every imaginable kind of exotic parasitic disease has been identified in our country. Parasites are an insidious public health threat in the U.S. today. They are insidious because so very few people are talking about parasites, and even fewer people are listening. They are insidious because physicians do not suspect, and therefore do not recognize, classic symptoms.

I was totally amazed to learn from *Guess What Came to Dinner* how parasites are the great masqueraders. Some of the symptoms of parasitic involvement are constipation, diarrhea, gas, bloating, irritable bowel syndrome, joint and muscle aches and pains, anemia, allergy, skin conditions, granulomas, nervousness, sleep disturbances, teeth grinding, chronic fatigue, and immune dysfunction. However, the most common symptom is *no symptom at all.*

About six months ago I was watching one of the late night talk shows and one of my favorite actresses and singers of all times, the Divine Ms. "M," Bette Midler, was talking about all the weight she had recently lost. She said that she had been sick for about four months and it was discovered that she had a parasite in her intestinal system. She did not go into all the details of symptoms, just that she could not eat. She joked about how all her friends wanted to know *where they could get one!* All kidding aside we don't want to get a parasite for weight loss or for any other reason!

Of course, the first place your mind wants to go with this information (after the shock wears off) is: "How can a parasite or worm live in my body without me knowing it is there?"

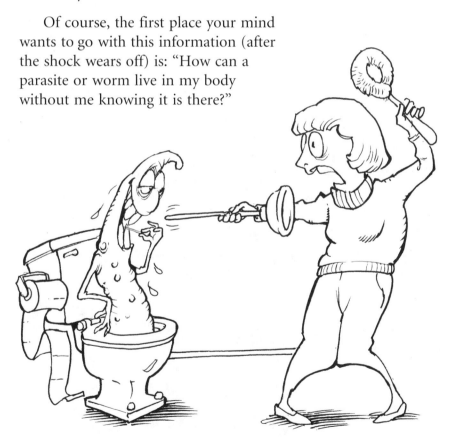

According to nutrition expert, Ann Louise Gittleman, ND, M.S., CNS:

Unfortunately, many of us suffer—or know people who do—from mysterious maladies that affect our feeling of well-being and for which neither we nor our doctors can find a curable cause. Some treatments or medications help for a while, but the condition never entirely goes away. We frequently continue to have sensitivities, intolerances or allergies to various foods, often accompanied by depression. Our bodies are telling us that something is physically wrong—but we are not listening!

SHOULD I GET TESTED FOR PARASITES?

In my opinion, you should save your money. If you are tested by a doctor for parasites (though chances are your physician won't suspect parasites in the first place), the results are most likely to come back negative. Does this mean that you are free from parasites? Unfortunately, medical testing procedures (besides being expensive) detect only about 20% of the actual cases of parasites. Dr. Ross Anderson makes this very valid point: "Of more than 1,000 species of parasites that can live in your body, tests are available for approximately 40 to 50 types. This means doctors are testing for only about 5% of the parasites and missing 80% of those. This brings the ability to clinically find parasites down to 1%. Now, if I had a 1% chance of winning in the stock market I don't think I would invest."

Parasites are THE most unsuspected source of ill health and suffering on the planet today. Make no mistake about it; nearly 8 out of 10 Americans are carrying one or more "uninvited guests" somewhere in their bodies.

– Anne Louise Gittleman, ND, MS, CNS

Another point to consider is that only 30% of parasites are living in the lower intestinal tract. The other 70% of the parasites, living in tissues, organs, and muscles, are undetectable in a stool sample.

With the statistics being what they are, save your money on all the fancy-schmancy testing, and just assume that you do have parasites. Get out of denial, realize that you are probably not one of the 5% of the population not infected with parasites (unless you've been living in a protective bubble all your life), and follow a simple herb program. End of story. Let's not make this any more difficult than it has to be.

Do you have:

- Gas, bloating, or burning sensation in the stomach?
- Unclear thinking and forgetfulness?
- Itchy ears, nose, or anus?
- Female problems with PMS and menstrual cycle?
- Male sexual dysfunction?
- Loss of appetite or lethargy?
- Obesity or trouble losing weight?
- More appetite than normal but still feel hungry?
- Grinding teeth while asleep?
- A craving for sugar?
- Bed-wetting?
- Drooling while sleeping?
- Blurry or unclear vision?
- Chronic fatigue syndrome?
- Cancer?

Anne Louise Gittleman, ND, MS, CNS, sums it up well: "If you have been suffering from symptoms you simply cannot get rid of with even the best diet, exercise, or stress relief program, chances are, parasites are the underlying cause."

SOURCES OF PARASITIC INFESTATION

How has this parasitic epidemic taken place? A quick look at the means of transmission of parasites will give us some answers.

Airborne. Remember, we all have to breathe. (Don't deny it: I've seen you.) Some parasites are airborne and you can breathe them into your body.

Food/restaurants. Have you ever eaten in a restaurant? You could be exposed to parasites. Improper washing of foods or the food handlers' hands can cause parasite infection. After I read *Guess What Came to Dinner*, a book about parasites by Anne Louise Gittleman, ND, MS, CNS, I was so paranoid I wouldn't eat in restaurants for months.

- ◆ Raw fish, sushi, or sashimi, and undercooked fish carry fish tapeworms.

- ◆ Raw beef and rare steaks or hamburgers carry beef tapeworms, toxoplasmosis, and possible trichinosis.

- ◆ Raw lamb can carry sheep tapeworms and toxoplasmosis.

- ◆ Raw pork carries pork tapeworm, toxoplasmosis, and trichinosis.

According to Gittleman: "In the *New England Journal of Medicine*, researchers have reported finding a new parasite that is transmitted to humans from fish. The Eustrongylides worm had been thought to be found primarily in fish-eating birds. In the case reported in the journal, the 24-year-old student complaining of severe pain in his abdomen underwent surgery for appendicitis. The surgeons found a normal appendix. They also found a 10-inch pinkish-red worm, which crawled out onto the surgical sheets. The student was a once-a-month sushi and sashimi eater and most recently had eaten sushi at a friend's home." (*Guess What Came to Dinner*, 1993.)

(After reading this, becoming a vegetarian is sounding better all the time!)

Gittleman identifies the factors which have contributed to the parasite epidemic:

Water. In California, for example, the Sierra Nevada waters are contaminated with giardia lamblia, an amoeba. This water travels down to the Bay Area and often contaminates the local drinking water, especially with cysts (parasites lumped together into balls) which may not be filtered out at the water plant. Home water filtration units should specify that they filter out cysts. Rivers and lakes may be contaminated with amoebas and protozoa. Swallowing water when swimming, skiing, kayaking, etc., can be another source of parasitic infection.

Day care centers/institutional care. Imagine that a day-care employee unknowingly gets fecal matter under her fingernails while changing a baby's diaper. She washes her hands very well (though she may not have used antibacterial soap), then changes another diaper or two, or ten. She can very easily infect herself and other children by passing parasites from one child to another.

Other people. People who are infested are another source of infection. Parasite cleansing programs should be done by the whole family, not just one member. Sexual contact and certain sexual practices (better de-worm your spouse or significant other) may also spread parasites. We are not just talking condoms here. You can contract parasites just from kissing your partner.

Traveling abroad. We used to think that parasites were a third-world-country problem, but in a "global village" formed in part by widespread international travel, parasites are a fact of life everywhere, even in your home town.

Animals/pets. Owning and living with pets involves many opportunities for parasitic infections. You must become very conscious of poop-scooping in your yard, using antibacterial soaps after cleaning up or touching your pets, scrubbing under your fingernails, etc. Washing hands after handling pets is a very important habit to instill in children. 90% of cats have toxoplasmosis. Cuddling up to your cat places you at as great a risk as does emptying its litter box. Wearing a mask when cleaning out cat boxes will prevent breathing in the cat litter dust and ova (eggs), but you'll have to use your own discretion when it comes to cuddling.

I know you love your dogs, but let's avoid swapping doggie saliva. Dogs can carry tapeworms in their mouths. When I see a child, or even worse, an adult, allowing a pet to lick their face and mouth while kissing them in return (even in the dog food commercials), it makes me nuts. I absolutely want to scream. I am serious. It is not cute, it's insanity. Please! I mean, puh-leeze! Do not, under any circumstances, allow or encourage your children to let pets lick their face or share their food. You know the ol' "let the dog and child share the ice cream cone" scenario. (Of course, after reading the last chapter on children you won't be letting them have ice cream cones anyway, right?) Please emphasize the importance of proper cleansing of hands and face after handling pets.

Let's really be blunt here (you should be used to that by now): *Should you allow any creature that has just licked its anus to lick a bit of food off your plate?* I mean, come on. Unless you use special sterilization techniques, simply washing the dishes (even in a dishwasher) isn't going to cut it. *The average dishwashing liquids do not kill parasite eggs.* You might as well drink out of a toilet. Of course, the obvious prevention is to de-worm your pets on a regular basis with parasitic herbs, but also to have the utmost cleanliness with them. A little paranoia over parasites and your pets will feel better too.

When I first read *Guess What Came to Dinner* (Gittleman, 1993) I just about flipped. I had known about parasites for

We have a tremendous parasite problem right here in the United States — it's just not being identified.

– Peter Weina, Ph.D., Chief of Pathobiology,
Walter Reed Army Institute of Research

years, but knowing and "knowing" are entirely different things. I went on a week-long cleaning frenzy that included every square inch of my house and pet quarters. I was an advocate for rescuing abandoned pets from animal shelters, cleaning them up, and finding them homes. So I was especially paranoid about what parasites these animals (bless their little homeless hearts) were bringing into my family's living environment. I was bleaching dog runs and pet dishes and blankets like you would not believe. (Bleach kills parasites and eggs.) My husband's chin hit the floor when he saw me flying through the house like the proverbial white tornado, disinfecting everything (and I mean *everything*). I would have thrown our bed mattress and box-spring in the washing machine if I could have made them fit! I bleached every nook and cranny imaginable. I consider myself a very fastidious housekeeper, and the thought of parasite dust floating around my house just made my skin crawl.

I did that for a while, then I took a deep breath and calmed down. You can't live in a plastic bubble or disinfect everything before you or your family touches it. I can only speak for myself here, but God forbid that I would not keep pets (they are a true joy in my life) for fear of parasites. Instead, I chose another solution. Later in this chapter are some natural ways to keep you and your pets protected from parasites.

WHAT YOU ABSOLUTELY HAVE TO KNOW ABOUT PARASITES

You must educate yourself. Ignorance is not bliss with this epidemic. I have actually had people squirm in their chair, or make awful faces when I even suggest how parasites may relate to their health challenges. The typical comment is something like, "I don't wanna hear about it." One man said, "What would it hurt if I don't know? What harm can parasites possibly do? We all have them, don't we?" I calmly replied, "They can kill you." I may sound overboard on this, but all passions are strong. I must emphatically state to you that *parasites can and will cause diseases that can lead to your death or the death of someone in your family.* Saying anything less than that would be professionally irresponsible on my part.

PARASITES CAN EAT HUMAN BODIES

There are two major categories of parasites:

Large parasites. These are primarily worms (large enough to be visible with the naked eye). Some worms can be 10, 12, or even 15 inches long and in most cases cannot travel to other parts of the body except the digestive tract. In *The Essentials of Medical Parasitology*, Thomas J. Brooks says: "Tapeworms are among the oldest parasites of the human race. Indeed, some species have become so well adapted to live in the human intestine that the host [man] may be entirely asymptomatic."

The fish tapeworm is the largest of the human tapeworms, reaching a length of 33 feet or more. There can be 3,000 to 4,000 segments in a single worm. One worm can produce more than 1,000,000 eggs a day. Dr. Bernard Jensen's book, *The Science and Practice of Iridology*, contains a picture of a 20-foot-long tapeworm passed by a patient who had absolutely no idea she was infested.

Smaller parasites. Mainly microscopic in size, these include protozoa and amoebae. Despite their near invisibility, they can be very dangerous. Don't take their small size lightly. One type of a tiny parasite that infects the colon is called entamoeba histolytica. This type of infection can also be found in the liver, the lungs, and the brain. The disease form is called amoebiasis, and is often transmitted via contaminated food or water.

According to Ann Louise Gittleman, once worms or parasites are established in the body, these invaders do the following:

1.   Worms can cause physical trauma to the body by perforating the intestines, the circulatory system, the lungs, liver, and so on. Put quite bluntly, parasites can turn your organs into Swiss cheese. When chyme is released into the perforated intestines, it then oozes into the lymph system. Some parasites invade the body by penetrating the skin, producing dermatitis.

2.   Worms can also erode, damage, or block certain organs. They can lump together and make a ball, or cyst. These parasitic cysts—particularly if they are located in the brain, spinal cord, eye, heart, or bones—produce pressure on these organs due to their size and weight. Obstruction, particularly of the intestine and pancreatic and bile ducts, can also occur. I mention in Chapter 17 that a parasite-cleansing program must be completed before attempting to detoxify the liver and gallbladder. This is very important because if the bile ducts get plugged or blocked with worms, then the gallstones cannot be released.

3.   Parasites have to eat, so they rob us of our nutrients. They like to take the best of our vitamins and amino acids, leaving the rest for us. They grow healthy and fat while our organs and skin starve for nutrition. Many people become anemic. Drowsiness after meals is another sign that worms are present in the body.

4.   Parasites irritate the tissues of the body, inducing an inflammatory reaction on the part of the host. They destroy cells in the body faster than cells can be regenerated, creating an imbalance that results in ulceration, perforation, or anemia.

5.   Parasites depress immune system functioning while activating the immune response, eventually leading to immune exhaustion. Certain parasites have the ability to fool the body of the host into thinking that the worm is a normal part of the body tissue. Therefore, the body will not fight the intruder.

Gittleman goes on to say: "Parasites depress immune system functioning by decreasing the secretion of immunoglobulin A (IgA). Their presence continuously stimulates the immune system, leaving the body open to bacterial and viral infections."

6. The most important way these scavengers damage us is by *poisoning us with their toxic waste.* In other words, they poop in our bodies. Not only do we have to worry about our own poop, we have to worry about parasite poop, too. Each worm gives off a certain metabolic waste product, of which our already-weakened bodies have trouble disposing. The poisoning of the host with the parasite's waste is a condition called *verminous intoxication.* It can be very serious for the sufferer and it is difficult to diagnose. The host (that's you and me) now has to work twice as hard to remove both its own waste and that of the parasite.

In her books, *Cure for All Diseases* and *Cure for All Cancers*, Hulda Clark maintains that all diseases have their start with parasitic infestation and environmental toxins. Ross Anderson, MD, states, "It never ceases to amaze me, when I hear of an adult passing a worm in total surprise, that they could have had such a creature living inside of their body for possibly years."

"BEEN THERE, DONE THAT"

Let me tell you my own worm story. Of course I *do* have a worm story. I wouldn't challenge you with your own health issues if I didn't have my own. You probably already know much more about me than you ever cared to. Embarrassing as it is, here it goes.

A few years after my bowel cleansing events, I had been taking a lot of garlic and black walnut herbs for an anti-fungal condition (these herbs are also historically known for their anti-parasitic properties). Well, out of the blue, when I turned around to flush the toilet I saw this 6-inch-long white "thing" floating in the toilet. Again, I almost went into cardiac arrest in my bathroom. Was this what I thought it was? A worm? *Oh my God*, I'm thinking ... I fished it out of the toilet and took it in a jar to my herbalist friend Marene, praying that I was just overreacting or imagining things. We compared it to the ascaris parasite picture in her book and confirmed that indeed I had passed an ascarsis worm. Marene asked me if this was my specimen, because she said my face gave it away. I was as white as a sheet. I was in shock. I just passed a worm, and the proof (whether I liked it or not) had been floating in my toilet and visible to my very own eyes. My kids got a kick out of showing their dad when he got home. "Mom's worm in a jar!" Thank God they didn't want to take it to school for show-and-tell.

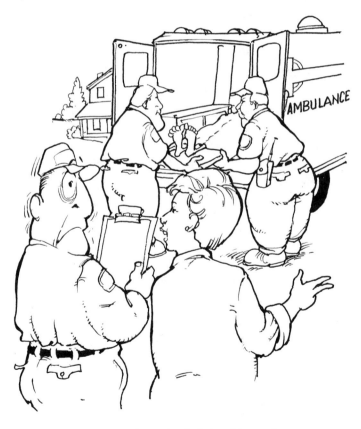

"My mom passed out right after she saw a large worm in her bowel movement"

Here is another true parasite story shared with permission from *The Herb Lady's Notebook,* as told by Venus Andrecht, herbalist, ID.

Helen's Hairball

My office door flew open. With a dramatic flourish Helen announced, "Venus, I passed a hairball last night!" She whipped a glass bottle from her purse and plunked it on my desk. I sat uneasily and eyed the bottle. Helen stood proud. A pleased grin broke out on her face. As my right-hand lady in the shop, Helen was pretty sure she knew what would delight me. Her short grayish curls danced. Nodding her head she continued, "I used to chew my hair in grammar school. I was real nervous, so I'd pull my hair around and chew on it all day. That was 60 years ago." She pointed proudly at the thing in the bottle. "That's a hairball." She gave a shudder. "I passed it this morning in my bowel movement. Pretty good, huh?" She looked at me, her thin body tense with expectation. She waited for my approval.

"Great," I said. "That's wonderful, Helen."

Helen sat down across from me and clasped her hands on my desk. "I did good, huh?" Her loop earrings with the stars bound and swung. "I figured you'd be happy with the hairball for your collection."

I slowly picked up Helen's specimen. I noted the pieces of tapeworm floating in alcohol, some nameless bits of something, and the so-called hairball. Strange. I carried the bottle to the front door where the light was better. Heck, I needed to be outside for this one. Helen trailed behind me. I held the glass to the morning sun. I turned it around and around again ... looked under it. Helen hung over my shoulder chattering about the old school days 60 years ago, and wasn't it a scream that after all these years a darn hairball would come out!

Suddenly I yelled, "Hey, look at that! This guy's got lips! My gosh! Look at that body! Helen, look at that body!" I turned around. No Helen. "Come here, Helen," I pleaded, "you've got to see this guy. Boy, you passed a good one."

I studied the fleshy creature more closely, my eyes squinting against the sun. It was about the size of a nickel. What Helen had thought was hair appeared to be made of stronger stuff, like hairy spikes. It made my skin crawl in a real fun way. After all, I hadn't passed it.

"Come on, Helen," I cried enthusiastically. "Where are you?"

Getting no response I turned and trotted back to my herb room. There was Helen lying flat on the couch. "Oh gosh," I said. I sat beside her.

She was pale. "I'm sorry," I ventured. "Maybe it's a hairball, Helen. I could be wrong."

Helen was silent. She stared at me blankly. "Yep," I soothed. "It's probably a hairball. It does look like a lot of hair there." I patted her hand. "Sure, that's what it is, a hairball. It happens all the time."

Helen stirred and looked hopeful. "You think so?" she asked.

"Oh yes," I answered. "That's it all right." I looked at her brightly and said, "And anyway, better out than in, right Helen?"

"Yes, I suppose so," she agreed.

"Tell you what," I said. "Why don't you just rest here a bit while I put some stock away." I gave her head a little rub and got up. "I'm sure it's just a lousy hairball."

"But I'll tell you what," I muttered quietly as I moved toward my shelves, "I never saw a hairball with *lips*."

❖ ❖ ❖

Following are two published articles warning the public of the threat of parasites.

Worms Outrank Cancer As Man's Deadliest Enemy

by Dolly Katz

Every year the American Cancer Society publishes the names of famous people, such as Duke Ellington and Jack Benny, who have died of cancer. This is done, the Society says, to serve as "a dramatic reminder of the full dimensions of cancer's human devastation."

When Abdel Halim Hafez, the most popular singer in the Arab world, died last year, his name did not appear on any list, although the disease that killed him causes more human devastation than cancer does. Hafez, 46, died from complications of schistosomiasis, an infection of parasitic worms that live in the intestines. Worldwide, an estimated 200 million people—equal to the U.S. population—are infected with this disease. And the schistosomiasis worm is only one of many parasites, ranging in size from microscopic single-celled animals to foot-long roundworms, which annually kill many more people than cancer does. The diseases they cause are as well known as malaria, and as obscure as kala-azur, which particularly affects children and is 90% fatal if untreated.

One out of every 4 people in the world is infected by roundworms, which cause fever, cough, and intestinal problems. A quarter of the world's population has hookworms, which can cause anemia and abdominal pain. A third of a billion people suffer from the abdominal pain and diarrhea caused by whipworms. Not much research is being done on these diseases. The U.S. spends more than $800 million a year on cancer research. All the nations of the world combined spend less that one-twentieth that amount studying parasitic diseases. As a result, there are no vaccines against them, and many of them are difficult or impossible to treat. There is no known treatment, for instance, for Chagas disease, a variant of African sleeping sickness that occurs in South and Central America.

But while these diseases occur predominantly in under-developed countries, the U.S. is not immune to them. Just about every parasitic disease known has been diagnosed in the U.S. in the last few years: schistosomiasis, trichinosis, giardiasis, toxoplasmosis, African sleeping sickness. Most, like malaria, are imported cases brought back by travelers. But a significant number are entrenched parts of our environment, kept alive in the U.S. by person-to-person transmission.

Take pinworms, for example. These parasites, which live in the lower intestine and rectum, are the most common parasitic infections of children in temperate countries. At least 1 in 5 children in the general population has pinworms. In institutions, the figure can go as high as 90%. All this doesn't mean that Americans ought to add parasites to the long list of disease we're supposed to worry about when we develop symptoms. But it's interesting and perhaps important to realize that to most of the world's people, cancer is as exotic a disease as sleeping sickness is to us.

– *The Miami Herald*, June 23, 1978

◆ ◆ ◆

Parasites More Common Than Believed, Study Says
by Ronald Kotulak

The first major nationwide survey of parasitic diseases has revealed that 1 in every 6 people studied has one or more parasites living somewhere in their body. The prevalence of these parasitic stowaways, which range from microscopic organisms to 15-foot tapeworms, has come as a big surprise, especially to physicians who receive little training in diagnosing and treating parasitic infections.

"We think of this country as a highly sanitized country," Dr. Myron G. Schulz said, "but that is not necessarily true. The large number of parasites means they are a cause in many diseases that baffle doctors. Many patients have experienced weeks of delay before the correct diagnosis was made and have been subjected to unnecessary laboratory tests, hospitalization, and even surgery," Schultz, director of the Parasitic Diseases Division of the Centers for Disease Control (CDC) in Atlanta, warned in an editorial appearing in an upcoming issue of the *Journal of the American Medical Association.* He said that the presence of parasites also means that many Americans are not as "clean" as they thought they were.

"What concerns me is that somewhere along the line there has been a breakdown in sanitation measures and people have ingested contaminated food, water, or dirt," said Dr. Dennis Juranek, assistant chief of the CDC's Parasitic Diseases Division. The survey pinpointed four problems:

1.   A parasite called giardia lamblia, which causes intestinal infections, is sweeping across the country. The parasite has now become the #1 cause of waterborne disease in the nation.

2.   Tapeworm infections appear to have increased by 100% in the last 10 years, an increase that may be linked to Americans' increasing fondness for raw or rare beef.

3.   Amoebiasis, the most deadly of the parasites, continues to be a serious problem, with recent outbreaks in South Carolina. Between 1969 and 1973 there were 242 reported deaths from amoebiasis, a microscopic organism usually passed from person to person.

4.   Illinois farmers are being plagued by a balatidium parasite from pigs that causes intestinal infections in humans. The survey involved examinations of 414,820 samples of feces in 1976. The examinations were performed by 570 public and

private laboratories in all 50 states, and the results sent to the CDC. According to the survey, 15.6% of the specimens contained one or more parasites. About half of these parasites are capable of causing disease. The large number of parasitic infections *discovered in the survey may not reflect the actual rate of infection in the general public, but it does reveal that the problem is much more widespread than most health professionals thought.*

"I'm sure that this high infection rate comes as a surprise to those who never considered parasitic diseases to be a major problem in the U.S.," Dr. Juranek said. The biggest problem uncovered in the survey was the high rate of infection with the giardia parasite. This parasite now appears to have spread to almost every state and is responsible for recent epidemics in upstate New York, Colorado, Washington, and New Hampshire.

This bug, a protozoan parasite, is microscopic in size and resembles a single-celled amoeba. The parasite coats the inside lining of the small intestine and prevents the lining from absorbing nutrients from food. Although not a killer, it causes illness characterized by diarrhea, weakness, weight loss, abdominal cramps, nausea, vomiting, belching, and fever. Most cases are misdiagnosed as bacterial infections, but unfortunately antibiotics have no effect on the parasite, Dr. Juranek said. Two drugs are effective in curing giardia: atabrine, an antimalarial agent, and metronidazole. Hundreds of small water systems throughout the county that do not adequately purify water may be contaminated with the parasite, according to Dr. John Hoff, an EPA research microbiologist.

Streams or watersheds may become contaminated through infected human sewage, and recent studies show that giardia-infected beavers may also contaminate water sources.

– Reprinted from the Chicago Tribune Service

◆ ◆ ◆

REMOVING PARASITES FROM OUR BODIES

Parasites are not stupid, and their sole goal in life is to live and reproduce at our expense. So how do we get these creepy-crawly parasitic creatures out of our bodies? Treatment of parasitic infection must be geared to eradicating the parasites rather than relieving the symptoms of infection. If the parasites are not eradicated, the infection will continue to cause untold damage to the system. Given a proper environment, a parasite colony can flourish to sometimes-fatal proportions. Our goal here is the removal of parasites from the system in conjunction with a bowel and gastrointestinal cleansing program. *Many parasites become embedded in the intestinal wall, and no herb treatments can effectively reach them until the mucous and encrusted waste matter overlying the worms are softened.*

The reason bowel cleansing is vitally important is that, as the parasites are dying off in our bodies, they give off very toxic and poisonous substances. To avoid reabsorbing these poisons into our system, the use of herbs, colonics, and cleansing programs such as the 7-day Boot Camp tissue cleanse and Loree's Bowel Blaster are essential.

So the protocol we want to follow is to:

♦ Build the immune system with herbs, vitamins, and mineral supplementation.

♦ Heal and cleanse the intestinal tract and bowel. This can be accomplished with herbal remedies. Sometimes the intestinal tract can be completely ripped up by parasites gripping into the intestinal tissue with their sharp teeth. Hookworms especially bite and suck on the intestinal wall, which can cause bleeding and necrosis (death of the tissue).

♦ Administer effective substances such as herbs, garlic, homeopathy, etc., to eliminate the parasites.

- Recolonize the gastrointestinal tract with friendly bacteria such as acidophilus, bifidophilus, etc.

- Follow a preventive program for prevention of reinfection.

Let's talk about some of the herbs that are historically used for parasitic infestation. Remember when I told you I was using garlic and black walnut hulls and consequently passed a 6-inch ascarsis parasite? Well, garlic has been used for centuries to treat parasites. Taken internally it is one of the most effective herbs for killing and expelling parasites. Garlic is effective against toxic bacteria, viruses, and fungus. It is known as the "poor man's penicillin." Garlic contains more germanium, an anti-cancer agent, than any other herb. Garlic has a detoxifying effect on all the body systems. It also has many other valuable properties for the body, but for the moment we will limit our discussion to its anti-parasitic properties.

Black walnut is most commonly associated with killing and expelling parasites, internal and external. Black walnut is effective on malaria parasites and on tapeworms. Black walnut also helps to burn up toxins, which can then be carried out of the body by laxative herbs.

Top nutritionist, Ann Louise Gittleman, has tried every parasite cleansing program, herb, and homeopathic on the market to get rid of these critters. Consistently, her clients report the most lasting results with the Verma and Para Systems for Uni Key (see Resource Guide) for general parasite removal. When you don't know exactly what you may be carrying, she recommends the Verma program first, followed by the Para program.

Verma-Key is for worms and flukes. The capsules contain black walnut, wormwood, balmony, wormseed, cascara sagrada, slippery elm, garlic and cloves. Verma Plus, a liquid tincture, is also for worms and flukes. It contains black walnut, worm-wood, centaury, male fern, orange peel, cloves and butternut. The Verma products are used simultaneously for about two months and then for about a week each month thereafter.

The two Para products for the one-celled critters like amoeba, giardia, blastocystits, and cyrptosporidium are Para Key capsules, which contain cranberry concentrate. The Para products should also be used simultaneously for two months and then for about a week each month thereafter.

After the parasites are removed from the system, Gittleman suggests a state-of-the-art general detox product called the Super GI Cleanse (available from Uni Key; see Resource Guide). This product is the best anti-parasite maintenance, because it contains mild anti-parasitic herbs for daily use and because it targets the liver, kidneys, lungs, as well as the intestines. Just remember to keep a plunger close to the toilet. You will be removing so much fecal matter after taking the Super GI, that it is best to be prepared. Gittleman told me she is thinking of having Uni Key provide a plunger with each Super GI order!

Another herbal product that I have been using for myself and my clients is Clear™. Clear™ is an ancient Mediterranean recipe that has been on the market for seven years. The results have been incredible. Clear™ contains green and black walnut, black seed, cloves, cramp bark, fennel seed, hyssop, pumpkin seed, peppermint leaves, gentian root, thyme, and grapefruit seed.

Clear™ is typically used in a 90-day program as a digestive and colonic aid. Clear™ is taken early in the morning with no food for 1 to 2 hours. (See Resource Guide, Chapter 24.)

A WORD ABOUT TAPEWORMS

The book, *Medical Parasitology*, by Markell and Voge, points out that therapy to remove tapeworms from the small intestine is only successful if the whole worm is expelled. If the head remains, the worm will grow back. My friend Marene and I heard, direct from the late Dr. Bernard Jensen, a way to remove tapeworms. This surefire method involves using warm milk and honey. You better sit down for this one. He said that the tapeworms will come out of the body, feel the cold air and break off, leaving the tapeworm head still inside. Since our goal is to get all (including the head) of the tapeworm we need to sit—yes, he said sit—(with your butt) in a pan of warm milk that has honey in it so the tapeworm will be drawn out of the anus. The whole tapeworm will come out of the anus because the warmth (of the milk) and the sweetness (from the honey) draw it out.

I assure you I am not making this up! I looked at Marene in total disbelief! I remember making some comment to her, like ... "Our clients already think we are a few clowns short of a circus. This suggestion will definitely cinch it."

Talking to other practitioners (and my clients) over the years I have heard many testimonials from people who have had worms crawling out of their eyes (tear ducts) and nose when starting a parasite cleansing program. Another client shares the experience of, after only two days on an herbal cleansing product, feeling a poking sensation in her lower abdomen and a wiggling sensation in one of her legs. The next day she passed an 8-inch worm, and since then has passed many different sizes and types of parasites. Are you still with me here? Hopefully you haven't thrown down this book and gone running for God knows where. This is important information you must hear. I've said I am a woman with a mission. Do you believe me now?

The 90-day Clear™ herbal cleanse is recommended twice yearly. Many people including myself choose to stay on a maintenance dose of 2 Clear™ capsules per day indefinitely for more vibrant health. We can be exposed to many things that affect our immune system, directly or indirectly, on a daily basis. If you have a lifestyle that exposes you to the possibility of such exposure, stay on a maintenance dose of Clear™, black walnut, or garlic.

Ann Louise Gittleman recommends the Verma & Para System (Verma Plus & Verma Key), an all-natural cleansing system designed to help eliminate intestinal worms. The Para System (Para Plus & Para Key) is a broad-spectrum natural cleanser used to help eliminate invasive microscopic parasites.

A word about parasite drugs or medications versus herbal programs. If you were given a prescription drug for a certain type of parasite, the drug would be parasite-specific. This means that it would kill only the parasite that it was designed for. You have read the statistics. Finding the type of parasite you are dealing with is like finding a needle in a haystack. Herbs, on the other hand, kill *all* types of parasites in the body. So wouldn't it make sense to just use an herbal program and keep this whole matter as simple as possible?

Remember, it is vitally important to treat the whole family for an infection or just for prevention. People who live together can infect one another when making food for each other, sharing bathroom facilities, kissing, being sexual, etc.

Remember, almost everyone has some form of parasites. The greater your illness and health challenges, the greater the number of parasites that could be living off you. So get passionate about getting rid of your worst enemy, parasites, and step up to the next level of vibrant health.

CHAPTER 15

■ ■ ■ ■ ■ ■ ■ ■ ■ ■ ■

Nature's Pharmacy

There are no known side effects from herbs used knowledgeably and wisely. Knowledge and wisdom are the key words. Herbs cannot be used indiscriminately, without knowledge, any more than food can. We must use common sense, fortified with a basic knowledge of the properties of herbs, in order to use them effectively.

– Stan Malstrom, *Own Your Own Body*

THE HISTORICAL USES OF HERBS

The history of herbs and herbal medicine is as old as the history of man. Herbal medicine has been a part of the history of every civilization of which we have record. Herbs have been used as food for centuries. Herbs are not like drugs; they produce no instant miracle cures. They work with the body, not against it. Herbs combined with good, sound nutrition and other natural modalities can cleanse and aid in strengthening and rebuilding the body. Herbs are a food. They act as food in nourishing the body. Herbs perform certain functions in the body, just as certain foods contain vitamins and minerals that help certain areas of the body.

Herbs can assist the body, rather than interfere with cleansing, elimination, and regeneration processes. Drugs, on the other hand, cannot regenerate cells and tissue. Synthetic drugs can also cause serious side effects. Then the body is forced to deal with drug side effects, as well as the disease process at hand. Herbs

The American Death Ceremony

It usually takes from 10 to 15 years; however, modern scientific advancements are shortening this period of time. It starts with one simple aspirin for a simple headache. When the one aspirin will no longer cover up the headache, take two. After a few months, when two aspirins will no longer cover up the headache, you take one of the stronger compounds. By this time it becomes necessary to take something for the ulcers that have been caused by the aspirin. Now that you are taking two medicines, you have a good start. After a few months these medications will disrupt your liver function. If a good infection develops, you can take some penicillin. Of course, the penicillin will damage your red blood corpuscles and spleen so that you develop anemia. Another medication is then taken to cover up the anemia. By this time, all of these medications will put such a load on your kidneys that they should break down. It is now time to take some antibiotics. When these destroy your natural resistance to disease, you can expect a general flair-up of all your symptoms. The next step is to cover up all of these symptoms with sulfa drugs. When the kidneys finally plug up, you can have them drained. Some poisons will build up in your system but you can keep going quite a while this way.

By now the medications will be so confused they won't know what they are supposed to be doing, but it doesn't matter. If you have followed every step as directed, you can now make an appointment with your undertaker. This game can be played by practically all Americans, except for the few ignorant souls who follow nature.

– By Dr. L.I., excerpted from *Roots of Disease*
by Stan Malstrom, ND, MT

have no known side effects, but, as previously mentioned, must be used with knowledge. Because herbs are very high in vitamins, minerals, and other nutrients that nourish the body, they may sometimes be used when the body does not accept food.

Although herbs are very effective in healing situations, they are best employed in the prevention of disease. Since the whole focus of this book is the prevention of disease, I advocate the use of herbs as nature's pharmacy to cleanse and regenerate the body. For the purpose of this book I will describe some of the most common herbs and herbal combinations used for detoxifying the colon and other organs, for removing parasites, and for regenerating the whole body.

HERBS

Alfalfa. The word alfalfa means "father of all foods." Alfalfa contains health-building properties. It helps our body assimilate protein, calcium, and other nutrients. Alfalfa has been called the king of plants because it is extremely rich in vitamins and minerals, including iron, calcium, magnesium, phosphorus, sulfur, chlorine, sodium, potassium, silicon, and trace elements. It is beneficial because of its vitality and nutrient properties; furthermore, the contents are balanced for complete absorption. Alfalfa is a body cleanser. It is high in chlorophyll and alkalizes the body rapidly. I personally consider alfalfa to be one of the most nutritious herbs you can take.

Aloe vera. This is one of the most popular and well-known herbs. Although aloe vera is widely known as the "first aid plant" for its soothing and healing properties externally, it can also be used internally in the gastrointestinal tract. Aloe vera can be used internally in an herbal cleansing program and as an aid in expelling pinworms.

Black walnut. Most commonly associated with killing and expelling parasites, internal and external, black walnut oxygenates the blood to kill parasites such as tapeworms, the malaria parasite, and ringworm. In oxygenating the blood it aids the respiratory system in cleansing the body. Black walnut has anti-fungal properties. This is what I was using when I passed that 6-inch-long "thing" (ascaris worm) out of my bowel.

Burdock. One of the best blood purifiers, burdock has been widely used to neutralize and eliminate toxins in the system. It can reduce swelling around the joints, and helps rid the body of calcification deposits by promoting kidney function, which clears the blood of harmful acids. It is best to use burdock in combination with other herbs, since it can start the body cleansing too rapidly if used by itself.

Cascara sagrada. Certain Native American tribes called cascara sagrada the "sacred bark." It is one of the strongest of the laxative herbs, promoting peristaltic action in the intestinal canal. It is one of the best herbs to use and is said to be non-habit-forming. Cascara sagrada helps the bowels function naturally and regularly from its tonic effects, and is very useful in cleansing the colon and helping to rebuild its functions.

Chaparral. With the ability to cleanse deep into the muscles and tissue walls, chaparral is a potent blood purifier. Chaparral is a potent healer for the lymphatic system and the liver. It is historically known as a strong antioxidant and antiseptic.

Chickweed. Valuable for blood toxicity. Chickweed is a mild herb that has antiseptic properties when exposed to the blood. It helps carry out toxins. Chickweed has been historically used to dissolve cellulite (fat) from the body.

Chlorophyll. Long called "nature's green magic," chlorophyll taken orally moves unchanged until it reaches the small intestines. Acting as an oxidant, it helps the body rebuild destroyed bowel tissue. Chlorophyll also helps the body eliminate mucous. It is a deodorant of the bowel wall, a natural antiseptic to the intestinal tract, and a blood builder.

Dandelion. One of the best blood purifiers and builders available, dandelion is rich in vitamins and minerals, especially calcium. This herb has also been used to build energy and endurance. When we are detoxifying, we need to support and pay attention to the liver. Dandelion benefits the function of the liver. It has the ability to clear obstructions, and stimulates the liver to detoxify poisons. It increases the activity of the liver and the flow of bile into the intestines.

Echinacea. This herb stimulates the immune response, producing white blood cells. It improves lymphatic filtration and drainage, and helps remove toxins from the blood. Echinacea, called the "king of the blood purifiers," is considered one of the best blood cleansers. It is often used in combination with other herbs.

Flaxseed. This natural laxative is soothing, and provides roughage with mucilaginous qualities. It heals the body as it nourishes, and is soothing to the throat, stomach, and intestinal linings. Flaxseed is used in many bowel cleansing programs.

Garlic. Known historically as an effective agent against toxic bacteria, viruses, and fungi, garlic stimulates the lymphatic system to throw off waste materials. It contains more germanium than any other herb. Garlic taken internally is one of the most effective herbs for killing and expelling parasites. Garlic should be in everyone's medicine cabinet.

Marshmallow. Best known for aiding the kidneys and bladder, marshmallow has been used historically to heal mucous membranes. It helps remove difficult phlegm and release the bronchial tubes while soothing and healing. It is a valuable herb for the lungs, where it helps remove mucous. It is a great healing herb for the gastrointestinal tract.

Peppermint. One of the oldest and most popular remedies, peppermint acts as a sedative for the stomach. It also helps strengthen the bowels and expel stomach and colon gas.

Peppermint should always be in the medicine cabinet. I always keep a very small jar in my purse as a breath freshener.

Psyllium. Considered an excellent colon and intestinal cleanser, psyllium lubricates as well as heals the intestines and colon. It does not irritate the mucous membranes of the intestines, but strengthens the tissues and restores tone. Most of us know the importance of psyllium as a bulking agent. However, there is a difference between the seed and the hull! Psyllium seed is wonderful for bulk. However, it is the hull that gives us the mucilaginous action that is so important to soothe and cleanse the colon.

Red clover. Red clover as a dietary supplement is valued for its high mineral content. A potent blood purifier, it is good for preventing health problems. Red clover makes a delicious tea and can be drunk freely.

Safflower. A natural digestive aid, safflower contains hydrochloric acid. It has the ability to remove hard sticky phlegm from the system and to clear the lungs. Safflower soothes and coats the entire digestive tract, helps heal the walls of the intestines and relieves intestinal gas. It also has a mild laxative action in the bowels.

Slippery elm. An amazing, mild-flavored, highly nutritious herb, slippery elm has the ability to neutralize stomach acidity and absorb foul gases. It acts as a buffer against irritations and inflammations of the mucous membranes. Slippery elm is a contact healer, both internally and externally. It coats and relaxes all inflamed tissues, including irritated and inflamed mucous membranes of the stomach, bowels, and kidneys. I have used this herb extensively with my clients, adding it to water to soothe the intestinal tissues.

Taheebo (pau d'arco). Obtained from the inner bark of the red lapacho tree that grows in the Andes of South America, taheebo or pau d'arco is considered the "everything" herb. You have to start slowly drinking pau d'arco tea; it is so potent it can give you a headache if you drink too much too soon. Start with half a cup a day and work up to several cups a day in a few weeks' time. Another good staple for the medicine cabinet!

Turkey rhubarb. Historically, turkey rhubarb has been used to cleanse the alimentary canal and the entire digestive tract. It improves digestion and appetite. Turkey rhubarb stimulates peristaltic action and glandular secretions. It is a good purgative for the intestinal tract.

Uva ursi. Used to strengthen and tone the urinary passages, this herb is especially beneficial for the bladder and kidneys.

HERBAL COMBINATIONS

All Cell Detox Combination, General Cleanser and Parasite Formula. All Cell Detox contains 17 herbs that support proper digestion and waste elimination. (gentian, Irish moss, goldenseal, marshmallow, fenugreek seeds, mandrake, safflower, myrrh gum, yellow dock, echinacea, black walnut, barberry, dandelion, St. John's wort, chickweed, catnip, cyani)

Artemisia Combination, Parasite Formula. Artemisia has a long history of use in China, Europe, and the U.S. for its antiparasitic qualities. The common belief is that artemisia contributes to an unfavorable environment for parasites. (elecampane root, mugwort herb, vegetable fiber, spearmint herb, turmeric root, ginger root, garlic bulb, clove flower buds, and wormwood herb)

Liver Cleanse Formulas. The liver is a filtering organ. This herbal combination helps the liver cleanse, heal, and function normally, and helps the gallbladder function normally. (red beet root, dandelion, parsley herb, horsetail, liverwort, birch leaves, blessed thistle, angelica root, chamomile, gentian, goldenrod, barberry bark, cramp bark, fennel, ginger, catnip, peppermint, wild yam)

Bowel Detox Combination, Intestinal System Product. Known for its tonifying effect in the colon, Bowel Detox has been called "colon aerobics." Many years of eating devitalized foods leave the bowel wall lazy and out of shape. This supplement is a must for any cleanse. Although it contains supplements besides herbs, it is included here because it is such a phenomenal product to support the intestinal system. [psyllium hulls, algin, cascara sagrada bark, bentonite, apple pectin, marshmallow root, parthenium root, charcoal, ginger root, sodium, copper, chlorophyllin, vitamins C and E (d-alpha tocopherol), beta-carotene, betaine HCL, bile salts, pancreatin, pepsin, selenium (amino acid chelate), zinc (gluconate)]

BP-X Combination, Blood Purifier Combination. These herbs help carry toxins away from the cells to the elimination organs, carry nutrients to the cells, and cleanse the blood and maintain health. (yellow dock, dandelion, burdock, licorice, chaparral, red clover, barberry, cascara sagrada, yarrow, sarsaparilla)

Clear™ Combination, Immune Formula. This is an ancient herbal recipe that has been documented as being used for over 600 years. Clear™ is an herbal combination currently used by physicians, health professionals, and colon specialists through-out the U.S. and Canada. (green hull/black walnut, black seed, cloves, cramp bark, fennel seed, hyssop, pumpkin seed, peppermint leaves, gentian root, thyme, grapefruit seed, and bee pollen)

CLT-X Combination. Soothes and cools digestive fires. Very calming, soothing, and healing to the intestinal tract, it coats the intestinal lining. (marshmallow, slippery elm, comfrey, ginger, wild yam)

Experience™ Combination, Intestinal System Product. This ancient herbal recipe is a digestive cleansing aid. It works well with Clear™ (described above) to promote proper elimination. It removes waste material, as well as mucoid material, from the digestive system and the rest of the body. (psyllium seed husk, rhubarb root, fennel seed, corn silk, King Solomon seed, kelp)

Herbal Trace Minerals Combination, Blood Builder. This is one of the best building combinations for the body, and three of the most nutritious herbs you can take. (alfalfa, dandelion, kelp)

Herbal Pumpkin, Parasite Combination. This herbal combination helps make the intestines inhospitable to foreign invaders. (pumpkin seeds, Culver's root, mandrake, violet leaves, poke root, cascara sagrada with hazel, mullein, marshmallow, slippery elm)

Intestinal Soothe/Build; also called UC3J Combination. This combination of herbs helps heal and soothe inflamed and raw tissue in the intestinal track. (chamomile flowers, marshmallow root, plantain herb, rosehips, slippery elm, bugleweed)

K & JP-X Combination. A diuretic, this formula helps cleanse, heal, and normalize the kidneys, bladder, and urinary passages. (juniper berries, parsley, uva ursi leaves, dandelion root, chamomile, marshmallow, ginger, goldenseal)

LBS11 Combination, Lower Bowel Combination. Combats constipation and supports proper waste elimination. Non-addictive, these herbs strengthen the colon and increase peristalsis. Normalizes the colon function. (cascara sagrada, buckthorn, licorice root, capsicum fruit, ginger root, Oregon grape, turkey rhubarb root, couch grass herb, red clover tops)

LH and Marshmallow/Fenugreek Combination. This formula helps expel mucus from the lungs and helps fight infection. It is best used with infection-fighting herbal combinations. (marshmallow, mullein, lobelia, slippery elm, chickweed)

Red Beet Root (formerly Fasting Plus). This formula is designed to replenish nutrients the body might need while fasting or during periods of weakness. The glands may require additional nutrients as the body uses energy stores. (licorice root, red beet root, fennel seeds, and hawthorn berries)

Small Intestinal Detox, Digestive Combination. A general digestive aid, this combination helps dissolve mucous from the intestinal wall. It also tones the small and large intestine. (marshmallow, pepsin)

U Combination. These herbs are "contact healers," and also stop bleeding. Adding slippery elm to this combination increases its soothing properties. (goldenseal, capsicum, myrrh)

Verma and Para Systems Combination. Used throughout the world, the Verma and Para Systems are the #1 choice of doctors, colon hydrotherapists, acupuncturists, iridologists, and health care practitioners. They are specifically designed to eliminate *all* stages of parasitic infestation (from cysts to larvae to full-fledged parasites) throughout the body, not just in the intestinal tract. (*Verma capsules:* black walnut, wormwood, balmony, wormseed, cascara sagrada, slippery elm, garlic, cloves; *Verma tincture:* black walnut, wormwood, centaury, male fern, orange peel, cloves and butternut; *Para capsules:* cranberry concentrate, grapefruit seed extract, artemisia annua, garlic, cayenne, slippery elm, bromelain; *Para tincture:* black walnut, artemisia annua, prickly ash bark, quassia, cloves and cranberry concentrate)

CHAPTER 16

■ ■ ■ ■ ■ ■ ■ ■ ■ ■

Real People, Real Stories

Some of the names and locations have been changed to protect the embarrassed! Any resemblance to anyone you know is purely coincidental. Some clients have chosen to enter the witness protection program.

For Pete's Sake, Read the Directions
(Another Ex-Husband Story)

One day when I came home from work (years after the bowel explosion disaster) my husband came up to me just panicked about the vitamins that had been caught in his throat and chest all day. He said these vitamins were like horse pills. Well, after hearing him whine for about an hour, I took him to the medicine chest to see what offending vitamins he was talking about. He pulled out a bottle from the cabinet and shoved it my face, saying emphatically "Here ... this is the bottle."

After looking at the label I could hardly contain my laughter. "Honey," I said gently, "these are the dog's vitamins."

"Oh my God," he gasped. *Maybe you will grow some fur in those bald spots*, I thought. I am telling you, if he started lifting his leg on our furniture, I would have taken him straight to the vet!

Another time I walked into the kitchen and stopped dead in my tracks. There was my husband taking all of his vitamins and herbs (which I had left for him) with a bottle of beer!

"Holy moly," I said. "Herbs and beer?" He just smiled at me, belched, and walked out of the kitchen.

◆ ◆ ◆

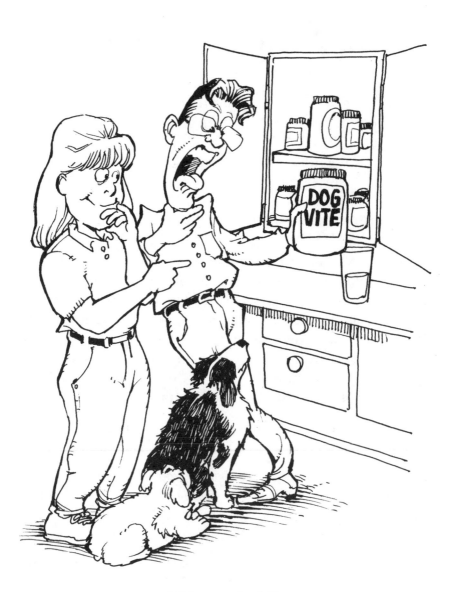

"Oh my God!"

J.C., San Jose, California
1/13/98

Dear Loree,

I am writing to let you know how much I appreciate you and the colonic treatments I have been receiving. After being a little skeptical and tentative in the beginning, I must say I have never felt better in my life. The Loree's Kick-Butt Bowel Blaster drink has done wonders for me. I truly feel that colonic hydrotherapy is the first step to becoming healthy. I would be happy to let you use me as a reference for any potential clients.

I want to share with you a true story about the Bowel Blaster drink that I think you and your readers will find amusing. I went to Tahoe with my friends for a bachelor party. I knew that I wasn't going to be taking your bowel blaster drink between shots, beers, and lap dances, so I decided it would be a good idea to take a *double dose* before I left. In the morning, after a hard night of poker and drinks, I got up to use the restroom. To my dismay the bathroom was occupied. I held on for as long as I could, when finally I urgently told the occupant in the bathroom: "Look dude, I'm about 12 centimeters dilated and about to give birth to a set of twins. Hurry up!" It ended up being triplets.

Thanks again Loree. I look forward to our continued professional relationship.

◆ ◆ ◆

Bill's Story

A friend of mine named Bill (he was one of the instigators of the Colonic Queen song) called me because he had an intestinal problem. Of course I had to razz him mercilessly because now he needed advice from the Colonic Queen. He was pretty humble when his intestines were giving him a bad time. Well, of course I would help him. He sent his wife Lynda over to get instructions and some herbs.

I wrote down the instructions very carefully. Included in this list of herbs were some capsules called LBS. I wrote down: Take 4 LBS capsules as directed. A short time after Lynda left my office I got a frantic call—I mean really frantic. "Loree," this panicked male raspy voice said, "Loree … this is Bill," (short gasp) … "You don't understand. I can't take 4 pounds of these herbs!"

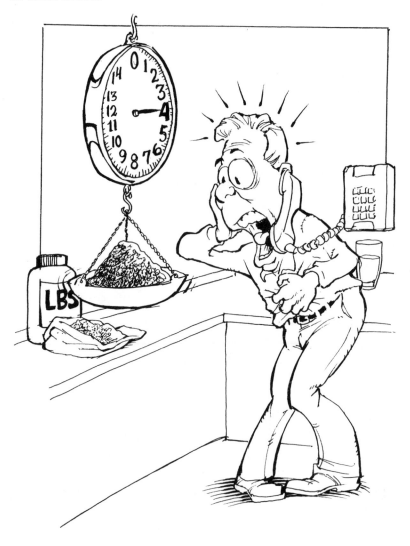

"Four pounds of herbs? Who said 4 pounds of herbs … Bill?"

"Well, you did, right here in the directions," gasped Bill.

When I realized the confusion, I just about fell off my chair in hysterics. "First of all, Bill, remember to breathe … No Bill," I said calmly, "take 4 of the LBS capsules—not 4 pounds!"

"Oh, what a relief!" he sighed.

The herb program did help him with his problem, and we got a lot of mileage out of this misunderstanding. Every time we saw each other he would say "Loree, I can't take 4 pounds of these herbs," and we would crack up laughing. It was our private joke for years.

◆ ◆ ◆

Here is another story, shared with permission from *The Herb Lady's Notebook*, as told to Venus Andrecht, herbalist, ID.

Cross Country Runs

Dan the trucker told me this one:

"I had a three-day run to make from San Diego to Texas. My chiropractor had given me some of your herbs. The ones to get rid of worms. You know, black walnut. Well, he told me to take 6 capsules a day, but I was going on this here run, see, and I knew I wouldn't take 'em on the road. So, I says to myself, make it easy guy. Take 'em all before you leave. So I did.

"The day I left, I took 18 of those babies all at once.

"The second day of the drive I noticed I was feeling a little uncomfortable. A little gas, you know. Pretty soon my guts started roiling mighty bad. Well, heck, I was steaming down the road here and no time to stop. I just lifted my rear a little to relieve the pressure. Pass some gas, right? Holy moly! I lifted my rear and whoosh! Splat! I passed more than air!

"It splattered all over the inside of my jeans and down my legs. I was horrified. Only it didn't stop there. Every time I let gas out it happened. By the time I saw a rest area I was soaked and mad as hell!

"I screeched my truck into that rest stop and was out the door and running. I shot into the bathroom. I musta' spent 2 hours there and another 15 minutes dunking my jeans and shorts in the toilet. Then, there I stood stark naked except for my shirt, shoes, and socks. I darted out the door with those damn jeans against my privates and scurried to my truck. Back on the road, I came to a weigh station. I told the guy in charge, 'Weigh the truck, I'm not getting out. Don't you dare ask why.'

"I had to drive 300 miles like that. Bare-assed."

◆ ◆ ◆

Narcolepsy

Gayle Marie Bradshaw
Sometime in 1977 . . .

Narcolepsy (när′-ke-lep-se): recurrent uncontrollable desire for sleep.

I stood there in his office, looking at an obese man sitting behind his desk, hoping he would have some answers for me. He was my neurologist. I had just finished a battery of tests, hoping to find out what was wrong with me. I couldn't believe what I was hearing. It was confirmed. Yes, I have narcolepsy. He pulled a pill bottle out of his drawer and said, "Here, take these and let me know how they work for you." I didn't attempt to reach for them so he got up out of his chair and came over to me. I was still in shock.

"I don't know what is the matter with you. Everyone has something wrong with them!" I looked up at him and thought,

I haven't taken drugs, an aspirin, a soda, junk food, sugar, or anything that I thought would harm my body since I was 22, and I am now 29, with four children under the age of 11 to support, and you want me just to take some pills that you know nothing about, and let you know how they work? I had hoped for more of an answer, something that would help me understand this disorder.

At least now I knew what I was dealing with.

I didn't know how to "fix" or cure it. Yet, during the past seven years I had recovered from many physical illnesses and disorders. At one time I was very ill, but once I learned about nutrition, food, sugar, vitamins, etc., I was able to turn my health around. I was considered a "health nut" by all my friends. I designated myself as my own family doctor. I took charge of my own health and the health of my children. But there I was, a single mother, no support from the dad, parents, etc. I couldn't be sick. Who was going to take care of us?

I knew it was only a matter of time before I would have a serious car accident, burn down the house by leaving the stove on, or not be awake when something tragic happened to my kids. I couldn't stay awake long enough to get through an hour, let alone the day. I was already having serious problems at the high-tech company where I worked in production. I would get lost walking to or from the bathroom, and fall asleep at my desk. I could drive for only about half a minute before I would fall asleep.

Many times I found myself waking up just in time to keep from running into a ditch or hitting another car. The kids would get up in the morning to get ready for school, and before I knew it I was waking up from a deep sleep. I would be terrorized. I didn't know how long I had been asleep, or where the kids were, or whether I had left something cooking on the stove. My God, anything could have happened.

I tried to get help from Social Security Insurance. But I couldn't stay awake in their office long enough to fill out the forms, and I couldn't remember my appointments or what documents to bring to my appointments. I finally had to quit my job. I didn't know about disability. I didn't want anyone to know I had a problem so I said I had a better job, and quit. I was on Aid to Dependent Children in between jobs. A lady in the employment office was so kind. She knew how much I wanted to work, and she did everything she could to help me find a job. I would find work, and I would be okay for the first few days. Because it was new it would work out. As soon as the job became routine, I would start falling asleep again.

I didn't take the drugs the doctor had given me. The day he gave them to me I took them to a friend who was a DA at the sheriff's department. He taught me how to use the *Medical Reference Dictionary*. He said, "If the information is written with regular print and the article is short, the item is somewhat safe. However, if it is written in bold or large print, it is not as safe."

When we looked up this drug, it had two pages of bold large print that said, "Warning: This drug is dangerous. Warning: Do not administer without medical supervision at all times. Warning: This drug depletes bone marrow."

The DA then said, "I am sure this is the same drug that killed my brother-in-law last month."

I didn't know what to do. I began to contemplate finding homes for my children. How was I going to be able to take care of them? Sharee was 5, Shane was 6, Brion was 9, and Kari was 11. But God helps all who ask. In 1980 I met a man, got engaged, and moved with him to Lake Tahoe, California, from Boise, Idaho. Together we tried to find doctors who might help me, with no luck. But at least I didn't have to worry about supporting my kids. He had a plumbing company in Tahoe and he began to teach me that trade. I would go to work with him, and learn what I could. But more days than not, I would find myself waking up in the seat of the truck, or underneath a house (yes, I crawled under houses with him), or not make it out of our house on days I was planning to work with him. I didn't have the stress of being a single mother anymore, but that didn't change my condition. I still couldn't drive, read, or sit still for more than a few moments without going into a deep sleep.

For those of us who have narcolepsy, when we fall asleep, we skip the first 2 stages of sleep and go deep into the 3rd stage. It isn't restful. I felt detached from my body. I had to teach my kids how to bring me back from this "place" I would go to. They would quietly talk to me, looking for a movement of my finger. This was the only way I could communicate. I didn't know where I was, but I knew I wasn't completely in my body like most people, so waking up was very difficult. The kids would look for a movement from my hand or finger, ask if I wanted to wake up, and then stay with me and gently talk to me until I could "come back." It was a very scary thing because I couldn't wake up unless someone came to help me. It was very difficult. Being married and not having as much stress in my life helped, but it didn't cure the narcolepsy.

Then, in 1982, a friend of mine sent me a colon cleansing product. She didn't know I had narcolepsy. Her husband was an iridologist and owned Nature Sunshine Herbs. I took them; they were awful. A few months later our family drove to Seattle, where my friend and her husband lived, and they taught me how to use the products. He did an iris reading for me, and then we returned home. I didn't have to worry about working and was fascinated with iridology, so I sent away for the correspondence course. During the time I was still taking the colon cleaning product. I wasn't sure if I would be able to get though the course, because it was so difficult for me to stay awake while reading.

But an amazing thing happened. What was supposed to be a one-year course, I finished in 6 weeks. I wasn't falling asleep. I was having problems with my marriage, and took the kids on a trip to Vernal, Utah. I drove 12 hours at a time, and stopped only because I was tired. I didn't fall asleep. Not once. I went to see a girlfriend and from there drove to Boise, Idaho, to visit family and friends. I then learned about a wonderful product called Barley Green. After a few days I drove 10 hours back to Tahoe. I was about 85 to 90% cured from narcolepsy. While I was taking the correspondence course, I learned about cleansing the colon with water. I bought a home-style system, called a Colema Board, which was wonderful. I truly believe that colon cleansing saved my life.

Why do I think colon cleansing saved my life? Let me ask you. If you only had a bowel movement once in 10 days, how sick do you think you would be? Since childhood when my mother questioned doctors about my constipation they said, "That is normal for her."

Do the math. Three meals *in* a day, one meal *out* in 10 days? If you or anyone you know has narcolepsy, share this testimony with them. This disorder nearly took my life. Today I have three grandchildren and a wonderful life.

◆ ◆ ◆

7/28/97
Linda Wood
Dana Point, California

Dear Loree,

For many years, my friends, family, and associates have told me I am "full of it," referring to my gregarious, outgoing personality. Little did I know they were correct in observing my condition.

I am writing to thank you for your referral to the Awareness Corporation and their products, Experience™, Clear™, and Harmony™. My less-than-desirable symptoms prior to using these products are too numerous to mention. However, the worst symptoms were chronic sinus pressure/headache, frequent diarrhea, depression, mood swings, and muscle and joint pain.

Within 48 hours of starting my cleansing program with Experience™, I was able to stop using over-the-counter decongestants for my sinus pressure and headaches. Also, within 48 hours, I started having solid stools — a great relief (no pun intended) after nearly 2 years of chronic constipation and the resultant diarrhea.

Nearing the end of my 90-day cleanse, I'm absolutely thrilled with the results I am seeing from these previously mentioned products. The best news of all, however, is your Bowel Blaster recipe. While the Experience™ digestive aid has helped tremendously, your formula is really moving things along quickly. I just wonder where all this stuff is coming from!

Thank you again and again for giving me back the ability to eat, sleep, and ... well, you know.

With much appreciation and affection ...

◆ ◆ ◆

M.B., San Jose, California

Up until 3 years ago (1997) I knew nothing about colon hydrotherapy. I had realized the importance of preventative medicine, and then learned that internal detoxification through colon hydrotherapy would be part of that regime.

I did have some concerns about my gas and bloating. I wanted to see if colon hydrotherapy would help with these issues. I am very fastidious with healthy eating so I just could not figure out what the problem was. I began seeing Loree regularly for colon hydrotherapy sessions. I did feel some immediate relief from the gas and bloating. Loree and a holistic chiropractor who specializes in nutritional modalities (and was very supportive of colon hydrotherapy) worked together to relieve my intestinal problems. I learned that in addition to the colon hydrotherapy I had to modify my diet to relieve my gas and bloating.

I was also amazed to learn the damage parasites can create in the intestinal system. We discovered that parasites were a contributing factor to my bloating problem. We left no stone unturned to get to the root of the problem.

Loree is so knowledgeable, straightforward, and direct with her information. I think she is truly amazing. During my colon hydrotherapy sessions I was able to learn, and to ask many questions about, how my body functions. I was able to gain a tremendous amount of knowledge in these sessions.

I think we all need to take responsibility and take charge of our health. We can't leave it up to doctors; it is up to us. I feel that we are each the president of our own health club. I believe we have to be very preventive in our actions. I can honestly say that I truly enjoyed my colon hydrotherapy sessions. I am very grateful that a treatment like this exists. I highly recommend colonics to anyone who wants to improve their intestinal, as well as their general, health.

Someone was kind enough to share this information about colon hydrotherapy with me and in turn I am glad to do the same. If sharing my experience will help educate others, then I share my story with all my heart.

◆ ◆ ◆

Here is another story shared with permission from *The Herb Lady's Notebook* as told to Venus Andrecht, herbalist, ID.

The Family That Cleans Together Cleaves Together

Let me tell you Carol's story. She's the Arizona herbalist who gave me the comfrey-pepsin cleanse. Like any good herb lady (or man) would, she decided to try the new cleanse on herself before foisting in on her friends. She took the herbs faithfully for some weeks, being careful to open the comfrey-pepsin and take it after her meals. When she had a bowel movement she would turn around and look. If you're going to do all that work, you want to know what you've accomplished. Right? One day, the same as any other day, when Carol turned around and looked, she screamed and fell back against the sink.

"Oh! Oh help!" she yelled. "I've passed a jellyfish!"

There in the toilet was a pale creature with a hump for a body. It slipped silently across the water. Carol lifted her head toward the ceiling and howled. Her husband and children came thundering up the stairs. They threw open the bathroom door. The jellyfish skittered across the water and dove to the bottom of the bowl. Her family screamed, Carol continued to scream. Most people can't continue hysteria forever, so eventually they calmed down and took a closer look.

Carol's brave husband fished out the jellyfish. They were puzzled to find that it was not a creature, but a large squarish piece of paper-like material. Apparently, as it slipped out of Carol, an air bubble had caught under the paper, giving it its movement and shape. When the bubble popped, the "jellyfish" collapsed to the bottom of the bowl. How exciting! Now you can see how herbs bring families together. That little group talked for weeks.

Marvelous things come out in a cleanse. One lady keeps a big stick by her toilet ... another a large silver spoon.

◆ ◆ ◆

Sept. 17, 1990
Jennie Munger
Hollister, California

I went to see Loree five months ago. I chose alternative and holistic therapy almost as a last resort. I needed help with a chronic digestive problem that was threatening to make recovery from an upcoming surgery a nightmare. My physician had pre-scribed medicine that would help on a short-term basis; I had used it many times before. I needed something that would be a lifelong answer, not a quick fix.

Loree listened to my concerns, asked questions about my lifestyle and eating habits, and asked what my long-term goals were as far as my health was concerned. She suggested a pro-gram of herbs and diet that I followed very carefully. I had only 5 weeks to get into better condition before surgery.

I had my operation, my recovery went beautifully, and I'm still using the herbs she recommended. I have never felt better, and my system has never worked as well as it does now.

What Loree has helped me accomplish, she has done for many other people that I know. I am grateful she is here and available to share her knowledge with others. I highly recom-mend her alternative and holistic therapy program.

◆ ◆ ◆

August 16, 1993

I want to give this testimonial anonymously because of my position in the community. I'm a registered nurse with 15 years of experience in nursing; 8 of those years were hospital nursing.

Because of the lack of ethics and competence which I have observed in the hospital setting, both as an employee and as a patient, I avoid standard medical care at all costs!

For 1½ years I had experienced ever-worsening constipation, extreme abdominal bloating, and incredibly foul gas that totally revolted my family. *It was bad!* I tried various over-the-counter and home remedies, but to no avail. At one point I had no bowel movement *whatsoever* for 2½ weeks. I felt terrible! Yet I knew that because I have good health insurance, if I sought help from a physician, I'd most likely end up in the hospital with every conceivable lab test being done for which the hospital could get reimbursement. Because surgery is a lucrative business, there was also a good chance I would end up with a colostomy. I decided that death would be better. So I did nothing; my family and I were suffering an intolerable condition.

After reading an article on bowel cleansing by Loree, I gave her a call. After following her recommendations for a month, I am no longer bloated or full of gas. Nor am I constipated. My personality is almost back to normal. I've been doing lots of reading on how to re-establish and maintain a healthy bowel and I am very grateful to have my health back.

Thank you, Loree!

❖ ❖ ❖

April 1998
Sheri, San Jose, California

What a delight. I just finished my first 7-day cleanse with Loree, and it was great. I had decided to do the fast while working and was surprised to find myself actually more productive than usual. The regularly scheduled cleansing drinks and herbs helped to keep my energy at a more consistent level than my previous eating habits did.

The nightly colonics were a lifesaver and I was amazed—okay, aghast—at how much material and toxins were released when I wasn't even eating. Seeing Loree each night helped to keep me motivated. She provided expert information and, best of all, helped to keep me laughing. I strongly recommend this cleanse to anyone wanting to re-commit to a healthy lifestyle. In just one week my skin has cleared, I feel light and energetic again, and I have already booked my next 7-day cleanse in another 7 weeks.

[Author's note: Sheri participated in the 7-day Bowel Boot Camp cleansing program mentioned in this book.]

◆ ◆ ◆

Another Bill

This is another true story ... different Bill. Bill and his wife were referred to me by a local veterinarian. Let me explain.

A local vet used to refer his four-legged patients to me for some additional nutritional help with herbs. Bill was quite skeptical of me and my herbal program for his dog. His wife convinced him to try it for the dog's sake. This guy was a Hollister cowboy right down to the fancy boots ... I really had to earn my credibility with him. His dog responded remarkably well to the nutritional program and Bill softened up to me.

After I gained Bill's confidence he shyly asked me if I could help him with a constipation problem. Me? Help with a constipation problem? Boy, had he come to the right woman! This guy had one of those big, hard beer bellies (an ol' poopy belly) whew ... we were going to have to do some work on this guy.

I told him if he drank my Loree's Kick-Butt Bowel Blaster Clean-Out-the-Crud Cleansing Drink religiously he would see some good results. Results? Boy, did he get results. He called me on the phone about 4 days later just ecstatic. He was so proud of the fact that he dropped 14 pounds of poop in just 3 days. He said (in his own words) that the toilet was full every time he had a bowel movement, which was about 4 times a day.

"Wow Bill, that is great news!" I told him. "See, I told you that Bowel Blaster drink would work . . . what do you think?"

"What do I think?" he said. "I think my wife was right! She always said I was *full of crap!*"

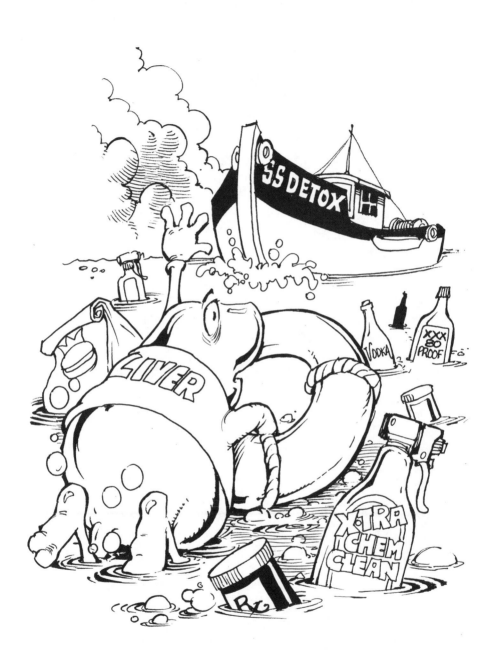

CHAPTER 17

■ ■ ■ ■ ■ ■ ■ ■ ■ ■

A Healthy Body Is a Clean Body

The road to health is the one that begins with an understanding and commitment to cleanse and detoxify the body, to restore balance, peace, and harmony. We must be willing to rise above selfish habits, realizing that the path of cleansing has implications for the intellect, emotions, and spirit. We need to accept our personal responsibility on this path.

– Dr. Bernard Jensen, Ph.D, ND

BETTER CLEAN ALL OF THOSE OTHER ORGANS, TOO ...

Even though we are primarily discussing the importance of the digestive system and the bowel, establishing optimal health is a team effort. A team of eliminative organs all work at the job of moving wastes and cellular material to the proper eliminative channels, to be excreted out of the body. Since the body is constantly breaking down or disintegrating, dead cells and other waste material must be eliminated efficiently. If eliminative organs are unable to function effectively (such as being hypoactive), the end products of metabolism as well as worn-out elements and cells will not be eliminated properly from the body. Think of how your kitchen would smell if you kept shoving food into an inoperable garbage disposal. The food would sit and rot, and not be broken down and removed.

Your body can eliminate up to 2 pounds of toxic waste daily through the skin, bowel, kidneys, and lungs. The body is only as clean as its eliminative organs.

THE SKIN

Our skin is one of the largest eliminative organs of the body and is sometimes called the third kidney. As mentioned previously your skin can assist the body in eliminating up to 2 pounds of toxins per day. We know that exercise and perspiration eliminate toxins through the skin.

I remember dancing with my husband and coming off the dance floor perfectly dry or, shall we say, in a "non-perspiring mode." My husband, on the other hand, was drenched. I remember our friends making jokes, asking us if he was the only one who had been dancing. Was I just standing there watching him? There was a distinct difference between his sweaty appearance and my non-perspiring, every-hair-in-place appearance. Yes, I was dancing, vigorously in fact, but it became apparent even in aerobics classes that I just did not perspire much. I have since come to learn that this is not a positive attribute and I am diligent in dry skin brushing to help my skin better eliminate toxins.

In an iris analysis it is vitally important to see if the skin is allowing toxins to be excreted. In iridology we look for a dark scurf rim (a thick, dark ring around the ring of the iris) to indicate hypoactive (underactive) skin that doesn't allow the toxins to be released from the body. Often in questioning a client with this scurf rim I find that the client does not perspire or sweat very much when they exercise. This type of person should be diligent in practicing dry skin brushing to remove the dead skin layers so toxins can escape.

DRY SKIN BRUSHING

One of the greatest gifts of health that you can give yourself is the gift of skin brushing. Dry skin brushing is one of the finest of all baths. No soap can wash the skin as clean as the new skin you have under the old. You make new skin on the body every 24 hours. The skin will only be as clean as the bloodstream. Dry skin brushing removes the top layer. This helps eliminate uric acid crystals, catarrh, and various other acids in the body. The skin should eliminate 2 pounds of waste acids daily. Keep the skin active. Skin brushing is the best way to get rid of the scurf rim found in the eye, which denotes an underactive, poorly eliminating skin. Dry skin brushing is also a highly effective technique for cleansing the lymphatic system. Because gastrointestinal cleansing softens hardened mucoid in the lymphatic system as well as in the intestines, performing dry skin brushing concurrently with a gastrointestinal cleansing program improves the skin brushing's effectiveness.

It is essential that the brush used contains natural vegetable bristles. You can purchase this type of brush at any health food store. Synthetic bristles should be strictly avoided. The brush should be kept dry and not used for bathing. When one performs dry skin brushing, the body should be dry, and the brush should pass once over every part of the body surface except the face. There should be no back and forth or circular motion, scrubbing, or massaging. One clean sweep does it. The direction of the brushing should be towards the heart. Start at the feet brushing up the leg and the buttocks. Brush up the hands and arms and down the neck and trunk. It is permissible to brush across the top of the shoulders and upper back, as the best contact with the skin is made that way.

Skin brushing should be performed once or, if desired, twice per day. A complete dry skin brushing takes no longer than 4 to 5 minutes and is highly stimulating and invigorating. I believe the best time to skin brush is before your morning shower. It would take 20 or 30 minutes of loofah or Turkish massage to get a similar effect. Just for fun, do this standing on a sheet of a dark color. You will be amazed at how much skin dust will be on that sheet. It is not uncommon for one's stools to contain large amounts of lymph mucoid a day or two after beginning dry skin brushing. This just represents an emptying out of the backlog of lymph mucoid present in the lymphatic system and has a lymph-purifying effect.

ACNE AND SKIN CONDITIONS

External skin conditions, such as acne, are a direct reflection of the toxicity and corruption going on inside of the body. Many of us have been conditioned to run to the pharmacy for the latest cream or lotion to give us clearer and more beautiful-looking skin. That money may be better spent on a colonic or some cleansing herbs than the latest external remedies and bottled promises.

A toxic body, especially the bowel and liver, can manifest itself with numerous skin conditions, not just acne. We must cleanse and detoxify the body at all levels, not just on the surface. One of the most important components of detoxification is the cleansing of the bloodstream. Your bloodstream is only as clean as your colon.

A number of herbs have been used historically for cleansing and purifying the bloodstream. Some of them are red clover blend, Oregon grape, burdock root, chaparral, pau d'arco, and an herb combination called BP-X. (See Chapter 15 for an expanded list of herbs and descriptions.)

When I was in Escondido at Dr. Jensen's ranch I heard the incredible story of a young man (in his 30s) named Michael. He had such severe psoriasis that his whole body was oozing and covered with red skin. In desperation, this man had traveled all over the world trying to find a remedy for his skin condition. His wife refused to sleep with him because his body was completely raw and oozing. At one point he was so hopeless about ever finding a cure that he tried to commit suicide. I don't remember how he got to Dr. Jensen's, but I believe everything happens for a reason. Michael's psoriasis condition was completely reversed through 7-day tissue cleansing and detoxifying the bowel. There are before-and-after pictures of Michael in Dr. Jensen's book on iridology.

Listed below are the suggested thought patterns that may coincide with certain skin conditions. (Louise Hay, *Heal Your Body*)

Acne. Probable cause: Not accepting the self. Dislike of the self. New thought pattern: *I am a Divine expression of life. I love and accept myself where I am right now.*

Skin. Protects our individuality. A sense organ. Probable cause of skin problems: Anxiety, fear. Old, buried gunk. I am being threatened. New thought pattern: *I feel safe to be me. I lovingly protect myself with thoughts of joy and peace. The past is forgiven and forgotten. I am free in this moment.*

THE LIVER AND GALLBLADDER

More than ever before in the history of mankind, human beings need to have healthy livers to break down the thousands of toxic chemicals that have insidiously crept into our environment and food chain. The liver is the gateway to the body and in this chemical age its detoxification systems are easily overloaded. Plants are sprayed with toxic chemicals, animals are given potent hormones and antibiotics, and food is processed, refined, frozen, and overcooked. All this can lead to destruction of delicate vitamins and minerals which are required for the detoxification pathways in the liver.

– Cabot, 1996

235

Typically, when I mention to my clients the cleansing actions of their liver and gallbladder, they are surprised and, quite frankly, have never thought of it before. Let's think about how your car would function if you never had an oil change. Your liver filters toxins from the body like the oil filter keeps impurities from your car engine. If my clients treated their cars the way they treat their bodies (and never provided any maintenance) they would all be walking for transportation. Just think of detoxification as preventive maintenance. Research suggests that at age 40 a person's liver is only operating at 30% capacity because of a 70% toxicity level. A healthy liver can deal with a wide range of toxic chemicals, drugs, solvents, pesticides, and food additives. Your liver also has amazing powers of rejuvenation, continuing to function when as many as 80% of its cells are damaged. Even more remarkable, the liver can regenerate its own damaged tissue. You owe it to yourself to detoxify and help your liver take a "deep breath" from these years of toxic abuse.

For many people, including children, another critical issue of the liver and gallbladder is that the biliary tubing can be choked with gallstones. Most people don't think about gallstones until they, or a family member, are signing an emergency surgery form when a full-blown gallbladder attack and life-threatening situation is at hand. At that point prevention is, as the saying goes, just too little too late. It would be like buying a smoke alarm after your house burned down.

In my opinion, cleansing and detoxifying the liver and gallbladder is one of the most powerful procedures you can do to improve your body's health. Many natural health practitioners (including myself) advise cleansing the liver twice a year. I firmly believe that if people would learn to cleanse their organs, such as the liver and gallbladder, emergency surgeries could be greatly reduced or avoided altogether. In her book, *Cure for All Cancers*, Hulda Clark states that you should cleanse until you remove 2,000 stones from the gallbladder. Just a note here: If you have had your gallbladder removed you still need to cleanse because the liver will make gallstones.

I want to be perfectly clear here that even though you do not have a perceived problem with your liver or gallbladder, it is still necessary to initiate cleansing and detoxification. If you are walking around the planet, breathing (I know you are ... I've seen you), eating (gotcha there too!), using chemical cleansing agents, soaps, drugs, etc., you need to cleanse your body's filtering system (the liver). Even though the liver has incredible regenerative abilities, we don't want it to become so exhausted that it loses its ability to detoxify itself. Many people will be shocked at what comes out of the liver and gallbladder, even when they don't have any diagnosed problems. I will have to add myself to this category. Here I go again with another one of my personal cleansing stories.

My first liver/gallbladder cleansing rendered me a jar half-full of green and tan gallstones, some as big around as my thumb. I was shocked. I put the gallstones in the freezer for a few months (to show some of my clients) with a warning to my housemates, "Loree's gallstones ... do not open."

At the time I did this liver/gallbladder cleanse, I had a male housemate who thought I was a lunatic. It was science vs. holistic healing in a clash of the titans. At one point we almost came to blows in the kitchen about scientific studies versus, in his words, my airy-fairy medicine. We were at opposite ends of the planet in our beliefs. You can imagine his reaction when he saw the gallstones in the freezer. The guy just about did a back flip in the kitchen (he was a tall guy and it was a very small kitchen) but hey, that was his problem.

Anyone who is around me for any length of time will learn that I have my cleansing cycles and rituals. I don't wear any strange clothing or go around chanting or anything, but many times I set aside social activities to complete a cleansing fast or a program. I take detoxification very seriously, despite being harangued mercilessly at times. I try not to be judgmental toward people with different beliefs. However, my days of flaming co-dependency and people-pleasing are over, and I don't have to justify my actions or my beliefs to anyone. I just follow my own path of consciousness. We all have the right to do what we feel is appropriate for our own body.

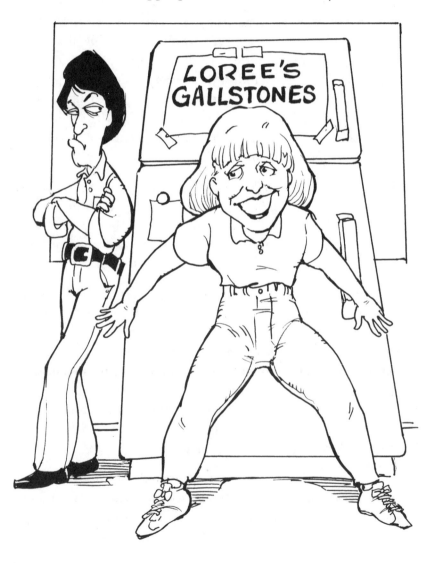

*Let no one presume to give advice to others who
has not first given good advice to himself.*

— Seneca

LIVER/GALLBLADDER FLUSH

This section provides the liver/gallbladder cleanse I used, based on Hulda Clarke's information, and that of many other herbalists. This is the most potent way to cleanse the liver. It can lead to much improved energy, a fantastically sharp mind, and a more efficient liver and gallbladder.

1. For 3 days drink as much apple juice as you can comfortably consume. Do not exceed one quart in a day. To each quart of apple juice add ¼ teaspoon of citric acid or orthophosphoric acid (obtain through a health practitioner).

   Alternate method: 15 drops of orthophosphoric acid, 2 times daily, for 2 weeks prior to the cleanse; and then 15 drops, 2 times a day, during the cleanse. (Check the strength of the orthophosphoric acid to determine that the above recipe is appropriate. Please consult your health practitioner.)

2. During this time concentrate on eating as well as possible: fruits, vegetables, nuts, seeds, and grains. Avoid animal proteins, except for fish.

3. On day 3 eat no fat for breakfast or lunch. After 2 p.m. on the third day consume no more solid food. Drink water and teas only. At 6 p.m. mix up 5 tablespoons of Epsom salts in 3 cups of water. This makes 4 servings of 1 cup each.

4. At 6 p.m. drink one ¾-cup serving. You may add ¼ teaspoon of vitamin C powder to improve the taste. You may also drink afterwards and rinse your mouth.

5. At 8 p.m. drink another ¾ cup of Epsom salts water.

6. At 9:45 p.m. pour ½ cup (measured) grapeseed oil or
    olive oil. (I personally can't stand olive oil and I prefer
    grapeseed oil. Many love olive oil and do well on it.)
    To this add ¾ cup of fresh grapefruit juice. Mix vigor-
    ously until watery.

7. At 10 p.m. drink the potion you have mixed. Lie down
    immediately. You may fail to get stones out if you
    don't. The sooner you lie down, the more stones you
    will get out. Be ready for bed ahead of time. Don't
    clean up the kitchen. As soon as you drink it down,
    walk to your bed and lie down flat on your back or on
    your right side with your head up high on the pillow.
    Try to think about what is happening in the liver. Try
    to keep perfectly still for at least 20 minutes. You may
    feel a train of stones traveling along the bile ducts like
    marbles. There is no pain because the bile duct valves
    are open, thanks to the Epsom salts. Go to sleep.

8. Upon awakening take your third dose of Epsom salts.
    Drink ¾ cup of the Epsom salts water. If you have
    indigestion or nausea, wait until it is gone before
    drinking the Epsom salts. You may go back to bed.
    Don't take this potion before 6 a.m.

9. 2 hours later take your fourth and last dose of Epsom
    salts water. Drink the last 1 cup. You may go back to
    bed.

10. After 2 more hours you may eat. Start with fruit or fruit
    juice. One hour later you may eat regular food but keep
    it light. By dinner you should feel recovered. Look for
    gallstones in the toilet with the bowel movement. Look
    for the green and tan kind since this is proof that they
    are genuine gallstones, not food residue. Only bile from
    the liver is pea green. The bowel movement sinks but

gallstones float because of the cholesterol inside. The tan stones are supposed to be really old stones.

You will need to release a total of 2,000 stones before the liver is cleansed. The first cleanse may rid you of the stones for a few days, but then stones from the rear travel forward. Sometimes the bile ducts are full of cholesterol crystals that did not form into round stones. They appear as a "chaff" floating on top of the toilet bowl water. Cleansing this chaff is just as important as purging stones.

> *This procedure contradicts many modern medical viewpoints. Gallstones are thought to be formed in the gallbladder, not the liver. They are thought to be few, not thousands. They are not linked to pains other than gall-bladder attacks. It is easy to understand why this is thought: by the time you have acute pain attacks, some stones are in the gallbladder, are big enough and sufficiently calcified to see on x-ray, and have caused inflammation there. The truth is self-evident. People who have had their gallbladder surgically removed still get plenty of green, bile-coated stones, and anyone who cares to dissect their stones can see that the concentric circles and crystals of cholesterol match textbook pictures of gallstones exactly.*
>
> – Clark, 1993

An important note: You can't clean the liver with parasites living in it. You won't get many stones and will feel quite ill. Parasites can also get stuck in the biliary ducts, so complete a parasite-killing program first before a liver/gallbladder cleanse.

TOXIC EMOTIONS

It is important to mention that organs in the body are associated with certain emotions. I once had a consultation with a male client and his wife regarding some health issues.

My analysis and muscle testing led me to ask this man, "What are you so angry about?" He was flabbergasted that I directly asked him that question with firm eye contact, but his liver (and some intuition on my part) led me down a different path than my original nutritional concerns. Our bodies speak volumes ... we just need to know how to listen.

Here are some thoughts from Louise Hay, *Heal Your Body:*

Liver problems. Probable cause: Resistance to change, fear, anger, hatred. The liver is the seat of anger, rage, primitive emotions, and chronic complaining. New thought pattern: *My mind is cleansed and free. I leave the past and move into the new. All is well. Love and peace and joy are what I know. I choose to live through the open space in my heart. I look for love and find it everywhere.*

THE KIDNEYS

According to the late Dr. Bernard Jensen, the kidney is one of the most abused organs in the eliminative chain, largely because most people do not drink enough water throughout the day. The kidneys must also accept toxic material from the liver, the bowel, and any other eliminative organs. During a fast or an extreme elimination diet, the kidneys are placed under additional strain from the intensified elimination of toxic material. The kidneys and the skin work together; as stated previously the skin is considered the "third kidney." So it would be reasonable to assume that if the skin were hypoactive (underactive) then it would put an extra burden on the kidneys. There's that team player theory again. If someone on the team is lagging (as my sons would say) then another team member has to pick up the slack. If perspiration is active, the kidneys don't have to eliminate as much toxic waste.

In my years as an iridologist I have seen many clients with an inherent weakness in the kidney area. So, regenerating the kidneys with proper diet, nutrition, and herbs is appropriate.

KIDNEY STONES

Kidney stones form when minerals that normally float free in the kidney fluids combine into crystals. When there is an overload of inorganic mineral waste and too little fluid, the molecules can't dissolve and they form sharp-edged stones. There are three types of kidney stones: those composed of calcium salts, the most common type (75 to 85% incidence); struvite, or non-calcium-containing crystals (10 to 15% incidence); and uric acid crystals (about 5 to 8% occurrence). It takes from 5 to 15 hours of vigorous, urgent treatment to dissolve and pass small stones. Anyone who has had a kidney stone "attack" will tell you it was one of the most miserable experiences of his life. Passing a kidney stone is rated right up there with childbirth in the pain department.

The little spikes or edges on the kidney stones cut like glass as the stones pass through the urethra, causing swelling, intense pain, and slight bleeding. One of the best ways to avoid kidney stone formation is to eat an alkalizing diet, emphasizing fresh fruits and vegetables, and avoiding excessive fat. Acid-forming foods should be eliminated from your diet: caffeine-containing foods; salty, sugary, and fried foods; and soft drinks that inhibit kidney filtering. As much as possible, avoid mucous-forming foods such as pasteurized dairy products, heavy grains, starches, and fats. This helps relieve and inhibit sediment formation.

Dehydration can also be a factor in kidney stone formation by creating a reduction of urine and a decreased rate of excretion of stone constituents. Be sure to drink plenty of water to assist the kidneys (all the eliminative channels for that matter) in flushing out impurities. It is suggested by herbalists to give your kidneys a cleansing at least twice a year. It is highly recommended to complete a kidney cleanse before cleansing the liver. You want to keep your kidneys, bladder, and urinary tract in top working condition so they can efficiently remove any undesirable substances incidentally absorbed from the intestine as bile is being excreted.

If it has been determined that you have some kidney weaknesses or have had kidney stones in the past, I strongly suggest that you have a sense of urgency about cleansing your kidneys. Below is a kidney stone flush that can also be used in a crisis.

KIDNEY STONE FLUSH

Drink the juice of ½ fresh lemon in an 8-ounce glass of water every ½ hour or until pain subsides. You can alternate lemon juice and apple juice.

- Take 3 capsules Kidney Activator Combination.
- Take Pain Combination (herbal aspirin if needed).
- Take 1000 mg. of vitamin C every hour.
- Take a warm catnip enema when pain subsides.
- It takes 5 to 14 hours to dissolve kidney stones.
- As a preventative, drink the juice of ½ lemon in a glass of warm water first thing each morning. Also, drinking cranberry juice and apple juice every day is beneficial to the urinary system.

Again, we need to look at toxic emotions to assist the body in its healing work. (Louise Hay, *Heal Your Body*)

Kidney problems. Probable cause: Criticism, disappointment, failure, shame, reacting like a little kid. New thought pattern: *Divine right action is always taking place in my life. Only good comes from each experience. It is safe to grow up.*

Kidney stones. Probable cause: Lumps of undissolved anger. New thought pattern: *I dissolve all past problems with ease.*

THE LYMPH SYSTEM

It is vitally important to assist the integrity of our immune system and eliminative channels by keeping the lymph system healthy. The lymphatic system removes wastes and toxins via a clear liquid that runs through lymph nodes and keeps our immune system healthy. The lymphatic system can be thought of as being responsible for waste disposal and immune response. Congestion and slow drainage result from excess wastes generated by an inefficient metabolism. The lymph system can become stagnant. The lymph system does not have a pump like the heart. Therefore, the fluid is moved through muscular contractions that "pump" the lymph. The best overall aid to a congested lymph system is exercise, which circulates the lymph fluid.

Get those tennis shoes on. Come on. I know you can do it. One, two, three, let's go ... *Exercise, exercise, exercise!* You get my point. Get out there and start moving, walk the dog, walk the cat, roller skate, jump up and down, I don't care what you do—just move and breathe. Being a couch potato will get you to the grave in a New York minute. Muscular contractions through exercise are the only way to keep the lymph system cleansed. So let's get moving!

> *Lymph congestion.* Probable cause: A warning that the mind needs to be re-centered on the essentials of life: love and joy. New thought pattern: *I am now totally centered in love and joy of being alive. I flow with life. Peace of mind is mine.*
>
> – Louise Hay, *Heal Your Body*

IT'S UP TO YOU

No one can do this for you. It's up to you to take responsibility for detoxifying as a preventive insurance policy for a long and healthy life. I think Nike said it best ... *Just do it!*

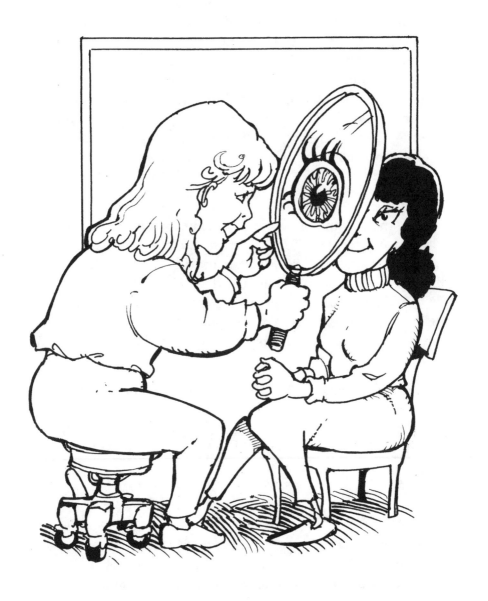

CHAPTER 18

■ ■ ■ ■ ■ ■ ■ ■ ■ ■

Iridology: What's the Bowel Got To Do With It?

Sit down before a fact like a little child, be prepared to give up every preconceived notion, follow humbly wherever and to whatever abysses nature leads, or you shall learn nothing.

– Thomas Huxley

IRIDOLOGY

As we approach the study of iridology (pronounced eye-ridology, not ear-idology) it will be helpful to keep an open mind and investigate the evidence presented by someone who was once a skeptic herself. My first experience of having an iridologist look into my eyes (see Chapter 1) left me speechless (and if you know me this is hard to imagine). I was so affected by that analysis that many years later I chose to further investigate the science and practice of iridology. For many years I have taken it upon myself to utilize iridology as a working tool to guide me with the nutritional and health needs of my clients and family. All I ask is that you stay with me here: I think you will find this subject as fascinating as I did.

HISTORY OF IRIDOLOGY

The following is the history of iridology, as related by Dr. Bernard Jensen:

In the early 1800s, a young lad named Ignatz von Peczely of Egervar, near Budapest, Hungary, caught an owl in his garden. The 11-year-old boy struggled with the frightened bird and faced its fierce claws as the bird instinctively tried to defend itself. In the struggle, the boy accidentally broke the owl's leg. As the lad and the owl glared at each other, the boy observed a black stripe rising in one of the owl's eyes. Von Peczely bandaged the owl's leg and nursed it back to health and released the bird, but the bird stayed in the garden several years afterward. Von Peczely observed the appearance of white and crooked lines in the owl's eye where the black stripe had originally appeared. The black stripe eventually became a tiny black spot surrounded by white lines and shading.

When von Peczely grew up, he became a physician and never forgot the incident with the owl. Working on the surgical ward of a college hospital afforded him an opportunity to observe the irises of patients after accidents, and preceding and following surgery. A study of the changes in the eye coincided with their injuries, surgery, or illnesses, and this convinced von Peczely that there was a reflex relationship between the various markings in the iris and the rest of the body. He was certain that the iris mirrored tissue changes of the various organs. Von Peczely created the first chart of the iris based on his findings.

Iridology has progressed tremendously since the 1800s. Numerous scientists and doctors have done research on iridology, revising and improving the iris chart. Iridology is based on scientific observation. It is the kind of science that cannot be related through scientific test, for it does not provide clinical information. The state of the art in Western medicine cannot reveal all the answers either. It is difficult to test one scientific system against another when two types of data are given.

The late Bernard Jensen, DC, Ph.D., internationally known as the father of iridology, pioneered the science of iridology in the United States. He developed one of the most comprehensive iris charts showing the location of the organs as they reflect in the iris of the eye. The iridology chart he developed (shown on the following pages) is still the most accurate available today.

WHAT IS IRIDOLOGY?

The eye has been described through the ages as the "mirror of the soul"; now we can see it as the "window of the body," enabling us to view indications of normal and abnormal states within the body and its organs. By way of definition, according to Dr. Jensen it is a science *whereby the practitioner can tell from markings or signs in the iris of the eye the reflex condition of the various organs of the body.* Iridology is the science of analyzing the delicate structures of the iris. Under magnification, the iris reveals itself to be a world of minute detail, a canvas with many features. The iris represents a communication system capable of handling an amazing quantity of information.

Dr. Jensen says many authors use the terms "iridiagnosis," or "iris diagnosis," but he prefers to use "iridology" because *the science of the eye is not the last word in determining the diagnosis of the patient* according to generally accepted methods and practice. It is one tool among many used in a good health management plan. This science can reveal inflammation, where it is located, and in what stage it is manifesting. Dr. Jensen categorizes the four stages of tissue integrity as acute, subacute, chronic, and degenerative (see the diagram on page 266). The iris reveals bodily conditions, inherent weakness, levels of health, and the transition that takes place in a person's body according to the way he or she lives. They say that success leaves its clues. So do destructive health and living habits. Iridology can warn a person of impending ill health and tissue degeneration, with the help of an iris analysis. It is an integral

Iridology Chart – Right Iris
developed by Dr. Bernard Jensen, DC

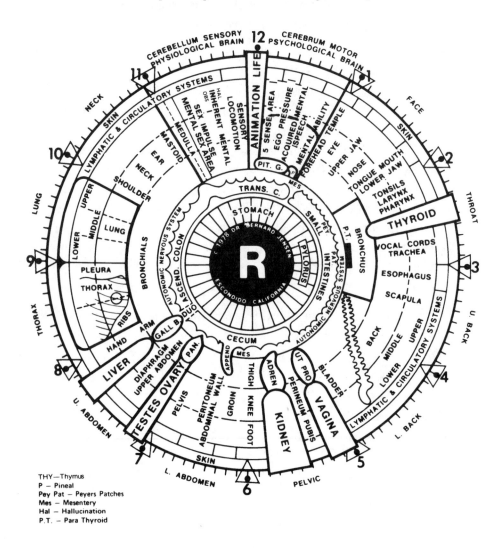

THY—Thymus
P – Pineal
Pey Pat – Peyers Patches
Mes – Mesentery
Hal – Hallucination
P.T. – Para Thyroid

© 1981 by Dr. Bernard Jensen, DC, Escondido, California
Used with permission of Dr. Bernard Jensen

Iridology Chart – Left Iris
developed by Dr. Bernard Jensen, DC

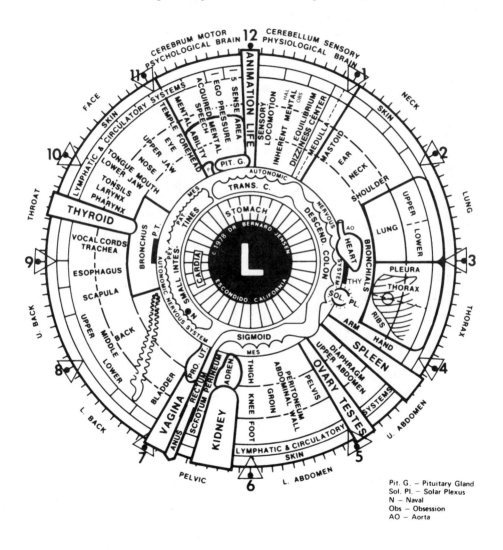

Pit. G. – Pituitary Gland
Sol. Pl. – Solar Plexus
N – Naval
Obs – Obsession
AO – Aorta

© 1981 by Dr. Bernard Jensen, DC, Escondido, California
Used with permission of Dr. Bernard Jensen

part of preventive medicine. The iris will alert us to the early signs of approaching disease.

IRIDOLOGY READS TISSUE

Iridology does not name diseases, but *it reads tissue integrity*. This is where iridology has one of its greatest uses: revealing weak tissue so that we can see tissue changes occurring before symptoms occur. This will reveal to the practitioner, doctor, and patient where, and what kind of, nutrition is needed for specific correction. In this respect, iridology becomes a powerful tool for preventable health issues and tissue rejuvenation. In my years as a health practitioner and educator, iridology has given me a powerful tool to help my clients with health issues that would have been less apparent without iridology.

A new female client came to me for an iridology analysis because she had some health concerns (we agreed that she would not share them with me prior to the analysis). In her analysis I became very concerned because she had extremely dark tissue (in a blue iris) in her breast area. The tissue was in the fourth stage of degeneration. I really agonized over how to approach this client with love, concern, and care. My fear was that she had breast cancer. As I stated earlier, iridology does not name a disease, but this is an example of how the breakdown of tissue integrity shows a possible disease process.

I gently expressed my concern over the breast area, trying not to alarm her, and recommended that she have an exam by a physician. Upon hearing my words she broke down in tears and told me she had, in fact, already been diagnosed with breast cancer in both breasts. She was checking out alternatives before deciding what to do. I gave her information on many alternative treatment options and offered her my support. This real-life drama was further confirmation of the potential diagnostic usefulness of iridology.

> *With superior knowledge the physician cures before the illness is manifested ... with inferior knowledge the physician can but attempt care of the illness he was unable to prevent.*
>
> – Ancient Chinese proverb

What iridology can reveal:

- The primary nutritional needs of the body.
- Inherently weak or strong organs, glands, and tissues.
- Constitutional strength or weakness.
- Relative amounts of toxic settlements in organs, glands, and tissues.
- Underactivity of the bowel.
- High-risk tissue areas in the body that may be leading to disease.
- Lymphatic system congestion.
- Poor assimilation of nutrients.

PRE-GAME SCOUTING OF YOUR OWN TEAM

The more information you have about your opponent, the better. Most good athletic teams prepare to take on another team by analyzing everything they do. They use a variety of techniques, including spying, in the search for one weakness, one chink in the armor. When they find it they try to exploit the living daylights out of it when the teams meet on the field. Your team is your body, mind, and soul, including all of your organs and tissues. Your supporting team members are health practitioners, physicians, friends, and family. Your opponent: disease and degeneration from the environment, food, alcohol, drugs, viruses, infections, etc.

The problem is, you have to know your own strengths and, even more importantly, your *weaknesses*. Do you think that opposing team won't search for the weakest link in your defensive setup to reach its own goal and beat you? What if you had a chance to see what your opponent already knows about you and is planning to exploit? You would know without a doubt all of your weakest points and be able to strategize a strong defense so your opposition could not get through. If your defense remains strong, and your weakest links are supported, you stand a better chance of winning the game.

Iridology gives you that pre-game peek at your own team's inherent strengths and weaknesses. Wouldn't it be to your advantage to shore up all your weak areas prior to your opponents implementing their strategy? How often have you heard a story about someone, maybe even someone you know intimately, who is going along in life and all of a sudden is diagnosed with a serious or terminal illness? That's what I mean about your opponent implementing their strategy before you can respond. Your opponent has known about your weakest link all along. A disease doesn't just develop overnight, where one day you are healthy and the next day you are given 6 months to live. Your opponent has been scrutinizing you, for many years in some cases, looking to tear you down at your weakest links (organs and body tissue). You are completely unaware of it—it is beyond your control, and you watch your opponent smugly capitalize and then drive in for a score.

What is your strategy now? Hopefully you will be a proactive and wise team player, carefully studying your own team's assets and liabilities. Iridology can help you with your scouting so you will come out the winner. A healthy life is a goal worth striving for, and it's a good idea to be armed with the best information possible to avoid being chewed up and spit out by the opposition. No one can play your game for you. It's guts and glory, or agony and defeat ... you get to choose.

> *No wealth accumulated in our lifetime can compensate us for the premature failure of our bodies.*
>
> – Floyd Weston, Nevada Clinic of Preventive Medicine

IRIDOLOGY AND THE BOWEL

Many of you are going to think that this is a real stretch—a relationship between the eyes and the bowels—but bear with me. Achieving insight into the digestive and the elimination channels of the body through iridology is such a gift. It is truly a remarkable discovery to realize that every organ is dependent upon the intestinal tract for nourishment.

In the iridology chart on pages 250 and 251, notice that the stomach is located in the middle of the iris immediately surrounding the pupil. Directly outside the stomach is the intestinal system (small and large intestine) and what is called the autonomic nerve wreath. These two "zones" are the hub of the body. This area is usually darker than the rest of the iris, and is where the greatest toxic accumulations are often found. By following the path of the wreath, it is possible to gather useful information about the tone, structure, and quality of the bowel, from which it picks up its nutrient supply. A slow-moving, toxic bowel spreads its toxic-laden contents to all body tissues.

When the bowel area shows many black dots and blackened portions throughout, this can be a sign of worms. Iridologists can often see long spokes coming out of the bowel area like spokes on a wheel. These are called radii solaris and indicate a slow-moving and toxic bowel. The individual needs to cleanse and detoxify his bowel and body. Often, but not always, *radii solaris* are an indication of parasitic infestation, or at least of an internal condition that is conducive to infestations.

It has been shown that there is a direct relationship between the large colon and corresponding reflex areas of the body (see

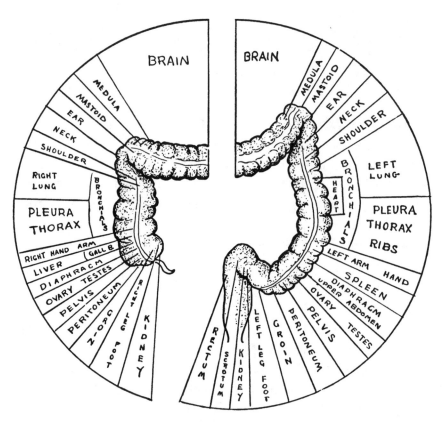

The colon produces reflex conditions in various organs in the body. In the above drawing, the organs opposite the particular part of bowel show what part of the body is affected by the colon directly. Symptoms in various parts of the body are relieved and many times eliminated when the intestinal flora have been changed. No matter what conditions we have in the body, it is affected by the bowel whether it is good or bad.

– Dr. Bernard Jensen, DC, *Science & Practice of Iridology*

illustration above). A problem in the colon produces a reflex symptom in the corresponding organ or tissue. Because it is a reflex organ, toxicity in the colon can affect the various organs as represented in the illustration. Due to the very close relationship between the colon and the rest of the organs, we should consider the extent to which the colon is responsible for the condition of any organ.

REFLEX ARC

When I was at Dr. Jensen's ranch he told a memorable story about the extent of the colon's impact on other areas of the body. He had a patient with torticollis, or "wry neck." For 5 days she had been treated mechanically by osteopathy, chiropractic, and physiotherapy, with no relief whatsoever. At first, Dr. Jensen thought it should be handled from a mechanical standpoint, by manipulation of the muscular and bony structures of the neck. Dr. Jensen's iris analysis revealed a focus of infection in the bowel at the splenic flexure (below the left ribs) which is opposite the neck (in iridology chart). Dr. Jensen questioned the patient about whether that "area" in the bowel had been giving her any difficulty. She stated that she had been sore there for months. She warned Dr. Jensen not to touch her there. When he further inquired if she had received treatment for this problem she said no one had suggested it. He then learned that she had not had a bowel movement for 7 days. With this information, a different approach was begun immediately. In a series of enemas, a great deal of extremely putrefactive material was eliminated, and within 3 hours she had almost complete relief from all neck symptoms.

I jumped on this theory with all my massage clients. I looked into the irises of everyone who would let me. I wanted to see if I could find a correlation between their bowel pockets (dark areas in the intestinal zone of the iris) and their physical complaints. The largest validation for this theory came when I tested the reflex arc with a patient in Dr. Ramsey's chiropractic office. The iridology analysis suggested a spinal and bowel correlation, which allowed me to confirm the area of the spinal column that was the patient's primary health issue. I would say my success rate was about 90%. He was amazed that the iris could tell so much.

Dr. Ramsey and I had a mutual male patient who had a chronic problem with his right shoulder. Dr. Ramsey was frustrated because chiropractic adjustments were not getting the results he was looking for. I also administered weekly deep tissue massage therapy treatments to this client with minimal results. Dr. Ramsey and I were both exasperated with our inability to secure adequate results.

I decided to check out this reflex arc theory that bowel congestion was at the root of this patient's shoulder problem. My theory was that if that were the case, cleansing the bowel would be necessary to help this patient with his shoulder problem. So I approached the patient and asked permission to scope out his eyes with a magnifying glass and penlight. To say that he was skeptical is an understatement. He thought I was downright weird. I pressed on and convinced him to just let me look, with the hope we would find an answer.

I did indeed find bowel pockets and toxicity in his iris correlating to the right shoulder. I tactfully explained to him how cleansing out the bowel would help his chronic shoulder condition. The man looked at me as if I just flown in from a spaceship and my hair was on fire. I think his comment was something like "What in the hell does my bowel have to do with my shoulder and zip it already with the eye stuff and just give me a massage." Needless to say this man was not open (I say this with no judgment whatsoever) to another avenue of healing. So Dr. Ramsey and I continued on with the same treatment, and the patient received the same mediocre results.

CONSTITUTION

One of the most crucial advantages an iridologist has in diagnosis is a peek at the inherent constitutional makeup of the client. I personally begin by looking at the constitutional character of the iris to gain an initial overall impression. Why start there? I always use the example of crocheting vs. knitting (bringing back fond memories of both my grandmas sitting in their chairs and crocheting). The closeness and uniformity of the fibers indicate a constitutional strength. In a knitted blanket, for example, the pattern of the yarn is very close together (with no space in between). This would indicate a stronger constitution. In the iris of the eye a strong constitution would be like the knitted blanket with the fibers tightly woven. A person with these characteristics rarely gets ill, responds rapidly to proper treatment, and recovers quickly.

By contrast, a crocheted blanket is loosely woven, with wider spaces between the fibers in the pattern of the yarn. The analogy to an iris would mean a person has a poorer or weaker constitution. The more irregular and open-spaced the fiber structure is, the more weakness is indicated in that body. Maintaining a high health level is more difficult for this body, and greater awareness of the forces and practices that enhance vitality is needed. A stronger constitution has a greater ability to retain nutrients, carry away metabolic waste, and carry on with life-giving cellular activities. A weaker constitution has more trouble maintaining nutrient levels; the metabolic process is slower, and toxic accumulations are more likely. Nonetheless, a weak constitution properly cared for can have good health and a long life. A strong constitution that is abused can be rapidly burned out and lost. Just as you can't change certain visible, genetic characteristics inherited from your parents—such as your mom's smile, your dad's gangly legs, and your height and bone structure (I have wanted to be tall and blonde all my life, but alas I have been 5'3" since the sixth grade)—you cannot change your inherited constitution. It's important to know what cards you were dealt, so you know how to play your hand, and you can support your body with nutrition to optimal health.

IRIDOLOGY: EYE TYPES

Iridologists have noticed that certain eye colors and eye types seem to be related to certain health tendencies. Following is an overview of these tendencies set out by eye types. So grab your flashlight and magnifying glass, and check out the ol' peepers in the mirror as you read along.

Blue eyes:
Lymphatic

Description: White collarette [autonomic nerve wreaths that are solid blue or gray-blue in color with no discoloration or psori (pigments)].

Tendencies: This is the "pure" blue eye found in people of European descent. It usually accompanies a classic phlegmatic disposition, which means the person is prone to lymphatic disturbances and catarrhal afflictions. This is probably due in part to the fact that people of European descent are frequently heavy consumers of dairy products. Blue-eyed people are also thought to have greater tendencies to accumulate uric acid in their bodies and to have kidney troubles. These people should pay particular attention to the following: mucous membrane areas (upper respiratory tract, bronchial, villi of lungs, digestive tract, and urogenital tracts), lymphatic tissues (tonsils, appendix, spleen, and lymph nodes), and membranes of the joints.

Common health problems: Common health problems for people with the lymphatic constitution include sinus trouble, sore throats, tonsillitis, earaches, bronchitis, asthma, swollen lymph nodes, skin catarrh (eczema and dandruff), kidney weakness, arthritis, and rheumatism.

Mixed eyes (greenish/hazel):
Digestive biliary

Description: Discoloration or psori (drug spots) on top of a blue-black background (fiber structure is visible through colon).

Tendencies: The blue-brown mixed eye has been linked by iridologists with a disposition toward biliary (bile-related) or hepatic (liver) troubles. It is believed that the coloration on top of the blue eye is a sign of toxicity in the body caused by digestive problems, especially when the pigmentation is concentrated around the center of the eye. Problems with the liver and other digestive organs can lead to further imbalances in the glandular and circulatory systems. These people should pay particular attention to their digestive system (stomach, pancreas, gall-bladder, and especially the liver) and their intestinal tract.

Common health problems: Health problems commonly associated with this type are hypoglycemia, PMS, indigestion, constipation, gas, toxicity of the digestive tract, anger, depression, difficulty getting to sleep followed by difficulty waking up in the morning, nausea, stiffness and achiness, headaches (especially migraines), food allergies, seasonal allergies, and candida.

Brown eyes:
Circulatory-hematogenic

Description: Pure brown eye with pigments covering iris fiber structure.

Tendencies: Pure brown eyes are difficult for iridologists to read because the pigment completely covers up the fiber structure of the eye. However, iridologists have noted some general characteristics of brown-eyed people. First, they appear to be predisposed to imbalances in blood composition and hence to blood disorders. It has been suggested that they have a possible inherent inability to store adequate supplies of minerals. They may especially have problems with calcium metabolism. These people should pay particular attention to their circulatory system (heart, blood, blood vessels), the organs that make blood (liver, spleen, bone marrow), the digestive system, and the endocrine glands.

Common health problems: Health problems commonly experienced by brown-eyed people include anemia, hardening of the arteries, all types of blood diseases, constriction and hardening of lymph tissue, possible reduced leukocytes in the blood, digestive troubles, mineral deficiencies, and early breakdown of the endocrine glands.

IRIDOLOGY: AN IMPORTANT ELEMENT

Used correctly, iridology gives an individual information concerning his health that is not available in any other way. Methods such as iridology should be investigated for their role in improving the performance of the body. While perfect health may not exist, we should work toward a more healthy way of living. Part of living a more healthy life involves proactive disease prevention. An iridologist's services are an important element in a comprehensive and holistic health care program.

CHAPTER 19

■ ■ ■ ■ ■ ■ ■ ■ ■ ■

The Healing Crisis and Hering's Law of Cure

A healing crisis is an acute reaction resulting from the ascendance of nature's healing forces over disease conditions. Its tendency is toward recovery, and it is, therefore, in conformity with nature's constructive principle.

— *Catechism of Naturopathy*

The healing crisis works on the principle of Hering's Law of Cure, which states: *All cure starts from within, out; and from the head, down; and in reverse order as the symptoms have appeared.*

"ALL CURE STARTS FROM THE HEAD"

What does that mean? To start with, it means a positive mental attitude is needed to become and stay well. It is the foundation of a healthy body. Clearing out mental and emotional toxins is as important as cleaning out the bowel, liver, or any other organ in the body. The person who nurtures resentment, hatred, anger, and other negative emotions sows the seeds of disease, not health. Such an individual will have difficulty healing.

I remember, as if it were yesterday, Dr. Jensen saying, "You can eat the best diet in the world, but if you have a miserable relationship or marriage you will not get well." This is not just referring to intimate relationships. It can mean all of our relationships and friendships. Do we have healthy, nurturing, loving relationships, or are we harboring resentments and unresolved anger? Do we scream and fight every time we are together? If you don't think this has an effect on your physical health … think again. We must scrutinize and evaluate everything that goes on in the mind as well as in the body.

Dr. Charm, a gastroenterologist in Walnut Creek, California, says that some of his patients have a case of "terminal seriousness," and that "a case of the sillies will keep away the ill-ies."

ORGANS WORK IN HARMONY TO CREATE A CRISIS

A healing crisis is the result of an industrious effort of every organ in the body to eliminate waste products and set the stage for regeneration. Catarrh (mucous) and other forms of waste that have been stored in the body are dissolved in a free-flowing state, and a cleansing, purifying process gets underway. Through this constructive process toward health, old tissues are replaced with new. A disease crisis, on the other hand, is not a natural one; every organ in the body works against it rather than with it, which is the opposite of any healing crisis. A healing crisis cannot be brought about without proper diet or fasting.

The experience of going through a healing crisis will seem very much like having an illness because one re-experiences disease symptoms. But there is an important distinction: elimination. In a healing crisis, bowel elimination is perfect. The bowel movement is natural, with all the eliminative organs doing their part. As a rule, the bowels do not work perfectly in a disease crisis.

In a healing crisis we develop fevers. When we have these crises, they appear to be the same as a disease crisis. They *appear* the same but they are different. A healing crisis brings on more

A healing crisis is really a blessing in disguise. Think of it as the whole body getting into action and correcting undesirable conditions. The good news is that your body is exchanging old tissue for new vibrant tissue. Dr. Henry Lindlahr said, "Give me a healing crisis and I will cure the disease." Hippocrates, "the father of medicine," said, "Give me a fever and I will cure the disease."

elimination through all five of the eliminative organs—skin, bowel, lungs, liver, and kidneys—than does a disease crisis.

The healing crisis usually lasts about 3 days, starting with a slight pain and discomfort which may become more severe until the point of complete expulsion is reached. During this time of crisis there is absence of appetite. One should follow the body's natural cravings. At this time the body needs water to help flush out the toxins that have reached the elimination point. This is a time for rest.

RETRACING THE DISEASE PROCESS

Remember that when a healing crisis is in progress you experience a temporary, acute stage of what previously occurred during the course of the disease. Eliminating the trouble involves a step-by-step retracing. As Hering's Law of Cure states: "All cure starts from within, out; and from the head, down; and in reverse order as the symptoms have appeared." This means your body will re-experience conditions and illnesses that were suppressed by drugs and that lie dormant in your tissues.

This retracing process makes sense when we consider that a person's living and eating habits in part determine the kind of tissue he has. In order to rid the body of tissue built up from injurious living habits—tissue that holds disease symptoms

265

Four Stages of Inflammation As Seen In the Iris

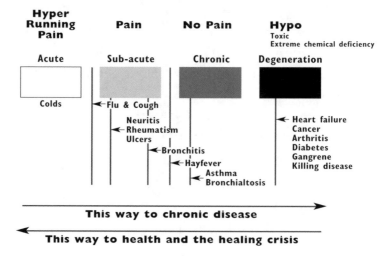

Hyper Running Pain	Pain	No Pain	Hypo Toxic Extreme chemical deficiency
Acute	Sub-acute	Chronic	Degeneration
Colds	←Flu & Cough		
	Neuritis		←Heart failure
	←Rheumatism		Cancer
	Ulcers		Arthritis
		←Bronchitis	Diabetes
		←Hayfever	Gangrene
		Asthma	Killing disease
		←Bronchialtosis	

→ **This way to chronic disease**

← **This way to health and the healing crisis**

Disease crises are developed when we produce chronic disease (traveling to the right).

Healing crises are developed when traveling to the left, away from chronicity and toward the acute stage of manifestation.

We build chronicity through suppression, bad habits, junk food, suppressive drugs, chemical shortages, enervation, poor circulation, and lack of the proper nerve motivation.

85% of diseases treated are chronic.

Hering's Law of Cure That We Follow in Getting Well

1. **Cure from within out ...**
2. **From head down ... and**
3. **In reverse order as disease had developed.**

Crises are found in hyperactive tissue. It is the will of that tissue to cleanse and purify or throw off toxic material in the body.

Health is earned, learned.
You get well when you're supposed to.

Used with permission of Dr. Bernard Jensen, DC

266

Inflammation is a reconstructive process and should not be suppressed. Every acute disease is a result of a cleansing and healing of nature.
— Henry Lindahr

lying latent in chronic tissue—the retracing process, i.e., the healing crisis, is necessary. You might be saying to yourself, "Why would I want to do all this work to get sick?" It may seem that you are sick, but old tissue is being replaced with new, healthy tissue, and you are actually preventing a disease process. It is absolutely essential to reclaim the health that you deserve through this healing process.

One experience that has always stuck with me is the story of Sylvia Bell, co-author of Dr. Jensen's book, *Tissue Cleansing Through Bowel Management*. When I was at Dr. Jensen's ranch in Escondido, California, he shared the story of how, while going through a tissue cleanse in her 50s, Sylvia had broken out with measles all over one side of her body. As a child, she had been given an anti-measles drug. When she got measles the drug had suppressed it into her tissues.

This is a perfect example of how the retracing process will produce original symptoms still dormant in the tissues. How could a woman re-experience measles at her age? By retracing the symptoms of the disease, that's how. Drugs just suppress all elimination processes and drive toxic material back into the body, causing it to be retained, which eventually produces chronic disease. We want to follow the natural laws of health and encourage elimination.

This is where I want you to stop and think about the habit of taking over-the-counter or prescription drugs for illness. Think especially about the effect this has on children. We, as a society, have gotten into the habit of giving children "something" every time they so much as sniffle. There are alternatives.

Consider finding a physician who is versed in herbs and homeopathy to treat your children. Children can be good sports about herbal remedies, once well-informed parents introduce them to the idea.

I have said this before, and I am going to say it again: *The body will do its healing work if we get out of its way.*

For certain life-threatening circumstances, taking drugs—such as antibiotics, for example—may be appropriate. But be really honest with yourself here. Most people take antibiotics for just about everything. We can't just blame doctors. Patients go to the doctor demanding a prescription for "this or that" instead of trying to work with the laws of nature.

TAKING RESPONSIBILITY

Where is our self-responsibility for our own health and the health of our children? Regrettably, some people seem unaware they are committing slow suicide every waking moment. They are not interested in their health until they lose it. Then they will pay anything to get well. That's when they start looking for something to remedy their condition. Health is learned, not earned. As we have discussed, disease takes many years to develop, and the return trip is not overnight. Health is a reward to the person who lives a better life with knowledge. We must be willing and committed to make the investment in ourselves for optimum health.

> *Our present system recognizes disease only when it has reached crisis proportions. This is tantamount to saying that a fire is only a fire when it has burst through the roof when, in actuality, it was a fire when the cigarette butt began to smolder in the rug.*
>
> – Carlton Frederics

CHAPTER 20

■ ■ ■ ■ ■ ■ ■ ■ ■ ■ ■

Powerpoopin'

LOREE'S KICK-BUTT BOWEL BLASTER
CLEAN-OUT-THE-CRUD CLEANSING DRINK

First thing in the morning, take 3 acidophilus/bifidophilus capsules on an empty stomach. Do not eat or drink anything for 20 minutes; this gives the acidophilus time to coat the intestines. We are attempting to restore healthy intestinal flora.

Note: Drinking coffee kills the natural bacteria in the intestines that we are trying to cultivate and restore. So, no coffee.

Also note: If you are taking the Clear™ product, your morning instructions will differ as Clear™ must be taken first thing on an empty stomach for best results. Caffeine diminishes the effectiveness of Clear™, so it must be avoided.

Cleansing drink, taken twice daily (morning and evening):

◆ 1 tablespoon liquid hydrated bentonite clay

◆ 1 teaspoon psyllium hulls combination

◆ 1 ounce of liquid aloe vera juice (if desired)

◆ Take this in 4 to 6 ounces of juice (drink quickly). Cranberry or grape juice are excellent choices.

◆ *Special considerations*—If you have an issue with blood sugar imbalances this would be too much concentrated sugar. Knudsen makes a juice called "Just Cranberry" with no sugar and only 14 grams of carbohydrate. It works very well with this cleansing drink. Or you can mix the cleansing drink with Ultimate GreenZone™, which will not elevate the blood sugar level.

Follow with 1 ounce of liquid chlorophyll in 8 ounces of purified water. (I call this the Chlorophyll Chaser.)

Herbs:

These herbs are to be taken twice daily, not at the same time as the cleansing drink. Usually one hour before or after the drink is fine. Try using half the dosage of the cleansing herbs for the first week until your body gets used to the laxative herbs, and then increase the dosage.

 ◆ Begin with 2 and increase to 4 Bowel Detox (used to restore peristaltic action)

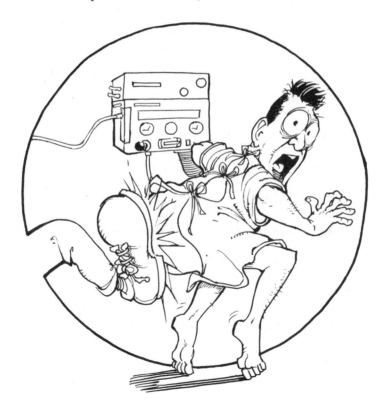

- Begin with 2 and increase to 4 cascara sagrada or LB SII (lower bowel stimulant and herbal laxatives). Please note: Use either LBS or cascara sagrada capsules with this program, not both. If you are prone to constipation, I recommend cascara sagrada.

Additional herbs may be added to your program to cleanse parasites, organs (liver, gallbladder, kidneys, etc.), lymph system, and the blood, and to re-alkalize the body.

- All Cell Detox (general digestive and cell cleanser)
- Liver formulas (for cleansing and building the liver)
- A liver and gallbladder cleanse may also be recommended in your detoxification program
- Herbal pumpkin seeds and black walnut hulls or tincture
- Garlic capsules
- Ultimate GreenZone™—a green superfood designed to build and alkalinize the body
- Digestive aid with all meals (very important)
- Food enzymes
- PDA Digestive Combination

Take 3 additional acidophilus/bifidophilus capsules before retiring. Here again, take them either 20 minutes before eating or 1 to 2 hours after eating. All other supplements and vitamins should be taken as usual and according to directions.

In order to get well, you must first go through the healing crisis. You must expect it, look for it, and work toward it.
— Dr. Bernard Jensen

What should I eat when on a cleansing program?

Foods to avoid while cleansing:

- Dairy products that are mucous-forming (milk, cheese, butter, etc.).

- Sugar in all forms (including alcohol).

- All junk and fast foods.

- Sodas and caffeine.

- Red meats, pork, fatty meats such as bacon.

- Fried foods.

Foods to increase while cleansing:

- Lots of pure water and herbal teas (at least a gallon a day).

- Fresh fruit and vegetable juice (invest in a good juicer and make your own).

During your cleanse:

- Eat lightly, such as salads (hold the goopy dressings) and soups.

- Keep starchy pastas and breads to a minimum or, better yet, eliminate them altogether.

- Don't overload the digestive system.

- Eat 5 to 6 small meals per day instead of 3 large meals.

- Light meats—chicken and fish.

I also suggest following proper food combining and natural hygiene as much as possible.

Please note: You are not being asked to fast on this Bowel Blaster program, only to revise your food plan.

CLEANSING INGREDIENTS

Here are some of the components of these two cleanses and the reasons they are essential.

First, the cleansing drink contains *hydrated bentonite clay*. Bentonite is ground-up volcanic ash found deep in the bowels of the earth (no pun intended). It is insoluble in water, but swells to 12 times when added to water. The molecules have two broad surfaces that have a negative electrical charge, while the edges are positive. Hence, bentonite can absorb or pick up many times its own weight of positively charged ions. Put simply, bentonite is like a magnetic sponge that removes toxins from the intestinal tract. Its action is entirely physical and not chemical. It helps to painlessly remove bacteria, parasites, and toxins from the entire intestinal tract. Since bentonite has such strong absorptive qualities, it may also remove some nutrients from the bowel, so the use of supplements is necessary on this cleanse.

Most of us know about the importance of *psyllium* as a bulking agent; however, there is a difference between the seed and the hull! Psyllium seed is wonderful for bulk; however, it is the hull that gives us the mucilaginous action which is so important for soothing and cleansing the colon.

Chlorophyll, long called nature's green magic, has surely lived up to its reputation! When taken orally in a liquid, it moves unchanged until it reaches the small intestines. Once within the cell of the bowel tissue, it acts primarily as an oxidant in the process of tissue production. In simple words, it helps the body rebuild destroyed bowel tissue. Chlorophyll also assists the whole body in its elimination of mucous by reducing the acid wastes. It's a deodorant of the bowel wall, a natural antiseptic to the intestinal tract. Bacteria find it difficult to live in the presence of chlorophyll, and therefore it is devastating to germs in the colon. Chlorophyll is a natural blood builder, with the same building effects as iron.

There are a lot of pros and cons about the use of vitamins on a fast. Remember, this is a cleanse, not a fast, and you must replace nutrients when using bentonite. I have found that vitamins mixed in an herbal base are especially beneficial. According to recent scientific studies in Europe, herbs act as a booster for the vitamins by helping us to assimilate them more easily. It's important to be selective about the type of multiple vitamin you purchase for your cleanse. Chelated organic liquid minerals have proven to be an excellent supplement for any cleanse.

The most abundant mineral found in the human body is *calcium*. Calcium aids the body's utilization of iron, activates several enzymes, regulates the passage of nutrients in and out of the cell wall, regulates the heartbeat, and helps prevent the accumulation of too much acid or alkali in the blood. Calcium is essential for the nervous system as a natural tranquilizer and as a sleep aid. It is a necessary addition to your cleanse.

Vitamin C (ascorbic acid) is one of the substances the body does not produce on its own. It must be obtained from the foods we eat and/or from a natural supplement. Knowing that the body cannot produce this important vitamin, we can understand why we have to add a vitamin C supplement to a cleansing program. Vitamin C dissolves mucous rapidly. Vitamin C on a cleanse can be in powder or the chewable form.

Certain herbs are especially helpful while on a cleanse or a fast. With weak adrenals, or when dizziness is experienced, licorice root and hawthorn help with stabilization, and at the same time keep the glands functioning better. The value of beet powder to aid in cleansing the liver and gallbladder is well known and widely used (for gallstones, too). Add fennel and you will be pleased to discover that gas, bloating, and cramping disappear. Fennel is also used as an appetite depressant. These herbs can be used alone or in combination.

Cascara sagrada has a long history of use for chronic constipation. This herb will move the bentonite and psyllium through the intestinal tract. Cascara aids the secretion of bile and increases peristalsis.

Ultimate GreenZone™. By combining protein-rich ingredients such as amaranth seeds, brown rice, millet, and spirulina with vitamin-rich food stuffs including carrots, broccoli, acerola fruit, and lemon bioflavonoids, Ultimate GreenZone is easily absorbed and metabolized into energy that you can feel almost instantly. Its fiber content helps your body maintain normal-range cholesterol levels and promotes bowel evacuation along with a healthy colon. It also provides digestive enzymes to support proper digestion.

7-DAY BOWEL BOOT CAMP CLEANSE

Remember I told you about my 7-day tissue cleanse where I dropped my colon lining? Well, now I am going to tell you about this cleanse. It is fashioned after a program developed by Bernard Jensen, world-renowned nutritionist and iridologist.

This 7-day program is designed to accomplish what we have been discussing — opening up the bowel to release its hardened contents so the rest of the body's tissues can then heal and regenerate. This program is a fasting cleanse where no solid food is ingested — just juices, cleansing drinks, herbs, and supplements. That is why I call it the Bowel Boot Camp: no whiners or sissies allowed.

For 7 days you consume a cleansing drink comprised of bentonite, psyllium, and liquid chlorophyll, 5 times a day (every 3 hours). In between the cleansing drinks you take precise amounts of herbs, supplements, and Ultimate GreenZone. You can make fresh juices and drink those if you get hungry, but no eating solid food. Let me emphasize that to you! You do not want your digestive system stimulated during this process.

You will not die from not eating for 7 days. Trust me, you will survive. Actually you will be completely surprised by how much energy you have without eating.

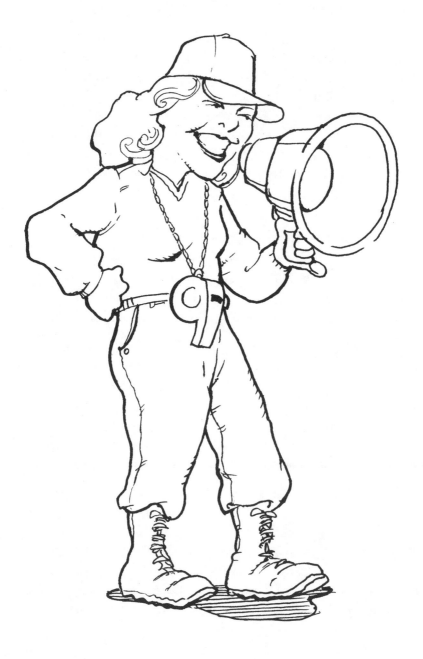

Instructions for the 7-day Boot Camp Cleanse

Five times during the day (every 3 hours):

- 2 tablespoons of hydrated bentonite
- 1 tablespoon of psyllium hulls
- Mix in 4 to 6 ounces of juice (drink quickly)
- Mix 1 ounce liquid chlorophyll in 8 ounces of purified water (the chlorophyll chaser).

Thirty minutes after the cleansing drink have one scoop of Ultimate GreenZone in 8 ounces of water with 2 capsules of spirulina.

Ninety minutes after the cleansing drink, take supplements listed below (5 times during the day):

- 2 laxative herbs (cascara sagrada)
- 2 red beet root formula
- 2 calcium magnesium (tablets or liquid)
- 2 multivitamin and mineral tablets or Daily Complete™ liquid vitamin and mineral supplement.

  (I personally recommend Daily Complete™. If you experience any nausea it may be from taking vitamin and mineral tablets on an empty stomach. To avoid nausea, you may need to take liquid vitamins such as Daily Complete™ during this cleanse.)

- Vitamin C tablet—100 mg.

Note: If you weigh under 140 lbs. Take cleansing drink and supplements just 4 times a day.

You are required to get a colonic at least once a day, and possibly twice a day if your situation warrants it. If you are using a Colema Board, take a Colema once in the morning and once at night.

At the end of the 7 days it is suggested that you take a supplementation (both orally and rectally) of acidophilus to restore all the good intestinal flora. The acidophilus should be taken orally for at least 30 days following this cleanse.

Points to remember during this cleanse:

- Be consistent with your drinks and supplements.

- If you get hungry or experience a drop in energy, take more Ultimate GreenZone with 2 capsules of spirulina.

- Drink lots of water to clear out toxins.

- You may have fresh vegetable juices (no canned or bottled juices).

- Dry skin brush every day to enhance elimination through the skin.

- The best exercise during this cleanse is walking every day and breathing in fresh air.

- Get plenty of rest and take good care of yourself.

Manifest an enthusiastic attitude. You are doing something absolutely awesome for yourself and your body!

FREQUENTLY ASKED QUESTIONS

What if I can't go without eating for 7 days?
Sure you can. You can do anything you set your mind to. Let me emphasize that to you! You will not die from not eating for 7 days. Trust me when I tell you that you will survive. You will probably be very surprised at how much energy you have without eating.

Can I exercise during the 7-day Boot Camp Cleanse?
Walking only.

If I do the 7-day Bowel Boot Camp detoxification program, how long until I drop the lining out?

I don't know. Our goal here is to expel this long ropy, snaky, black gunk as a result of this cleansing process. It took me five of these 7-day cleanses and 1½ years to get my colon clean. We have to have patience with our bodies. Remember, patience and persistence.

If I do the 7-day Bowel Boot Camp cleanse, how many colonics do I need to do?

A professional colonic once daily for the entire 7 days. If you are using a Colema Board, at least twice daily: one in the morning and one in the evening.

Isn't that a little excessive?

No! What's excessive is the buildup of poop in your intestines!

How many times a year should I do the 7-day Bowel Boot camp cleanse?

It is recommended that a 7-day cleanse like the 7-day boot camp cleanse should be done several times a year. If you have a stubborn health condition present this may warrant proceeding with this cleanse three to four times a year. I personally have done this cleanse once or twice a year for the last 17 years! I also fast one day a week and a few days a month (as discussed later in this chapter). My suggestion is that you discuss this matter with your health professional or colon therapist for recommendations on your personal health concerns.

How is Loree's Kick-Butt Bowel Blaster different from the 7-day Bowel Boot Camp Cleanse?

For those of you who are still cringing and whining at the thought of not eating for 7 days, I have thought of a way to still cleanse your bowel. That is why I designed the Loree's Kick-

Butt Bowel Blaster Clean-Out-the-Crud Cleansing Drink. Very simply put, in the 7-day Boot Camp cleanse you fast; on Loree's Bowel Blaster you don't. This drink contains the same products (in different proportions) as in the 7-day Boot Camp Cleanse, but you take it 2 times a day. You eat a modified diet and continue with your normal lifestyle. For dietary suggestions see the instructions in Loree's Bowel Blaster.

Which program should I do first?

My recommendation is to start with Loree's Kick-Butt Bowel Blaster program. Follow this program for about 4 to 6 weeks and you will have an easier transition into the 7-day Bowel Boot Camp Cleanse.

An important consideration involves the seasons. I recommend the 7-day Boot Camp Cleanse for between the middle of March and late October. Fasting during the direct winter months is harder on the body. You will find that you get very cold and chilled. If someone comes to me in, say, November or December, I would recommend that they stay on Loree's Kick-Butt Bowel Blaster program until spring, before embarking on the 7-day Boot Camp Cleanse. Keep this in mind, and time your cleanses accordingly. For more information on this theory, please read *Staying Healthy With the Seasons* by Elson Haas, MD.

How many colonics do you suggest with Loree's Bowel Blaster drink?

I generally suggest a series of 6 to 10 colonics at the beginning of Loree's Bowel Blaster program to really get things moving, because that is the point of all this effort: to blast that crud off the bowel wall, right? The colonics will help remove the fecal material being loosened up by the cleansing drink. Then I suggest a colonic at least once or twice a month for maintenance and to monitor your progress, which could take up to a year.

Can I work during these cleanses? Won't I have to stay near the bathroom all day?

You can work! Absolutely! I never took time off work when I did these cleanses. Just keep a lighter schedule, don't work excessive hours, and don't take on a lot of social engagements. Use common sense and get plenty of rest. Many people go away for a week or so to cleanse and I highly recommend this if your schedule and finances allow. (The Resource Guide includes a few listings of places like this, so you could pursue that if you wish). In the beginning of Loree's Kick-Butt Bowel Blaster you can have more copious bowel movements (remember the story of Bill) in the first few weeks or so, then these will taper off. Your body will be playing catch-up with your backup of fecal matter, but you will not have explosive, urgent diarrhea. I am not going to blow up your intestines (like I did with my former husband). Can you see it? News flash ... *wife kills husband with herbal bowel cleansing program ... film at 11 ... Oops!* This program is balanced with herbs that cleanse but that also retone and build the intestinal system. You will not have to camp out in the bathroom. See "For Pete's Sake, Read the Directions" in Chapter 16, and as long as you don't make those mistakes you should be okay! You won't be delivering bowel triplets or running from roadside rest stops half-naked, with your clothes tucked over your privates!

Will I get a lot of gas when I start to detoxify?

When cleansing the body of old fecal matter and eliminating parasites, gas and toxins can be produced. Many people who have probably been suffering from autointoxication (self-poisoning) their whole life will produce foul-smelling gases as old fecal material becomes stirred up and activated. I use the example of a pond. The mud settles down to the bottom and the water appears somewhat clean. When you walk through the pond it stirs up all the mud, and it becomes very cloudy and murky. Herbs stir up old fecal matter that can produce foul-smelling gas and bloating. As your body gets more cleansed, this will subside. Everyone in your household will become very excited when this subsides.

How long will it take until I completely clean out my colon?

That is the $64,000 question. The average person takes a year or more to cleanse out their colon. The average person has 10 or more pounds of impacted feces in their colon. I hope I can impress upon you that it is crucial to be patient and persistent with your body. Many of us have taken years to get into this unhealthy condition, and it cannot be undone in just a few weeks or months. I love Covert Bailey's (the fitness guru of *Fit or Fat* fame) response when asked by a client how long it will take them to get fit. His answer was: "How many pieces of string will it take to reach the moon?" There are so many factors that determine a person's state of health, it is hard to predict when a person's colon will be cleansed of old fecal matter. Clients always ask me how many colonics they will need until they are cleaned out. Heck if I know. I am not trying to be flip here, but how much milk did you drink, how many hamburgers or servings of macaroni and cheese did you eat in your lifetime? Do you get my point? The ultimate goal here is to drop that mucous lining whether it takes 10 colonics or 100. Commit to that goal and to whatever it takes for that outcome.

Will I see parasites when I get a colonic?

Chances are you will not see any parasites going through what is called the view tube of a colon hydrotherapy machine. The reason is that the material goes through very rapidly and it is really hard to determine what is what before it passes. Some colonic machines have a collection unit on one end so fecal matter can be collected to send in for parasite testing. Most parasites are microscopic and cannot be seen. Just because you don't see any doesn't mean you did not dislodge any during a colonic. They hang out in the mucous and sometimes come out in clumps.

I had a special friend, Bob, who was lending his butt (in the name of science) when I was getting my colon hydrotherapy training. I gave him a colonic and unbeknownst to me he had eaten mung bean sprouts in Chinese food the night before. I saw all these long stringy things that I thought were a mass of worms all tangled up, flying by in the view tube. I just about fell off my stool! He saw the shocked look on my face and after questioning him he told me about the bean sprouts. Boy, were we both relieved. One important note here is that I told Bob he needed to assist his digestion because those bean sprouts were whole and not digested. I also told him if he wanted to eat mung bean sprouts, great—but not before a colonic session (we had many laughs over this one).

Will colonics kill parasites?

Colonics will remove the mucoid matter that the parasites live in, but the water alone will not kill them. That is why herbal programs are essential in eradicating parasites and their eggs (larvae).

What do you prescribe to kill parasites?

I don't prescribe anything. Those words will land me in jail. I can only tell you what herbs have been used for historically (such as killing parasites, constipation, and rebuilding the body). I suggest several herb books in the Resource Guide. Study them, and make choices that feel right for you and your family.

Do I have to use your cleansing products, or can I use my own?

These programs have been designed to work synergistically. I do not recommend picking and choosing different supplements or herbs in the program. I will be pretty blunt here (are you surprised?). Either do the programs as designed or don't do them at all. Let me tell you why. If I gave you the recipe for a casserole and you left out some of the ingredients, it would not taste as good as if made correctly. These programs are designed the same way. If you take out the cascara sagrada, for example, and just do the cleansing drink, you run the risk of having your intestines bloat up because the psyllium does not have a laxative herb to move the bulking agent through the intestinal system. This is just one scenario. Everything in the program is there for a purpose: do not pick and choose.

First and foremost, work with a knowledgeable colon therapist. They will work with you and know your medical history and concerns. Many colon therapists have also designed their own programs with products they are familiar with and that work very well. Many cleansing products on the market are available through health practitioners (such as colon therapists) or health food stores. I recommend that if you use products suggested by your colon therapist, then follow their instructions carefully, stick with their program in its entirety, be committed, and be persistent.

I personally recommend using the herbal source companies suggested because I have worked with their products for many years and I can gauge their results. I also suggest that if you decide to use any of my programs, such as Loree's Kick-Butt Bowel Blaster, then please use all the products I have created in the program as directed. Also, inform your colon therapist of what products you are taking and show them my program.

Can I take parasite-cleansing herbs without cleansing my colon?

Absolutely not! People try to save money by buying only the parasite herbs and not the bowel cleansing or system-building herbs ... bad choice. Again, are you going to be serious about this or screw around? If you are taking parasite herbs without bowel cleansing (both herbal and external), you run the risk of all the parasites' toxins and excrement flooding in, then saying the herbs made you sick. The herbs only circulated the parasite toxins in your body. Follow the programs as designed to minimize discomfort.

I said it once and I will say it again: Follow the programs as designed, or don't do them at all.

Will the herbs make me sick?

The herbs won't make you sick, but the toxins being circulated in your bloodstream and lymphatics may make you sick. If you get sick it is because you brought it on yourself with incorrect eating habits, use of drugs, etc. Please review Hering's Law of Cure in Chapter 19.

Do you guarantee your bowel cleansing program?

If you want me to say that you will drop a big bucket full of black, snaky colon debris or bowel lining in 3 months, 6 days, and 5 hours, I can't. I can, however, guarantee that you will get out of the program what you put into it. If you approach this half-assed you will get half-assed results — it is up to you. If you are diligent with your program you will see results. I love the example I read about Oprah and her results in running a marathon. Someone was whining about how easy it was for her to train for the marathon because she had a personal trainer and a personal chef on staff. Her personal trainer, Bob Greene, said, "Oprah could not hire someone to get up at 5:00 every morning and run 6 to 8 miles for her. She was diligent in her commitment and training and deserves all the results she got."

What is your commitment level? The results depend on you. Only you can decide.

How can I get support during my cleanse?

If you decide to do the 7-day Boot Camp Cleanse and you want support, call IACT or Specialty Health Products (see the Resource Guide) and find a colon hydrotherapist to support you through this cleanse.

Is it really necessary to do external cleansing of my bowel during these cleansing programs (such as colonics, Colema Board, etc.)?

Go back and re-read this book!

SHOPPING AT THE HEALTH FOOD STORE

Many of you will just want to go directly to the health food store to get cleansing products. Even though my preference is to have you consult a health care provider, many of you may not be ready to take that step. I believe that some proactivity is better than just doing nothing. If you seem to fit into this category then my suggestion is that you develop a rapport with the staff in the nutrition department and learn from them. There are many detoxification products on the market and it is hard to know what is the best for you and your lifestyle. A caring and informed staff will go a long way toward helping you make the best decision for you and your family.

I will give you some suggestions on companies that I know have reputable products carried in your local health food store. I must honestly say that I have never personally used most of these products, but I am going on company reputation. Some of these products are packaged in a one- or two-week supply. As I have stated before, that is a start but there is no one-week solution for years of dietary indiscretions.

- ◆ My first and foremost recommendation is Sonne's #7 Hydrated Bentonite and #9 Psyllium Husks made by Sonne's Organic Foods (I have personally used this product).

- ◆ Nature's Secret – Ultimate Cleanse, Ultimate Fiber and Parastroy for parasites

- ◆ Gaia Herbs – The Supreme Cleanse Source Naturals Cleanse

- ◆ Source Naturals – system & essential enzymes

- ◆ Soloray – Total Cleanse

When considering a cleansing program please be sure to include a good acidophilus/bifidophilus culture to replace all the good bacteria in your intestinal system. One product I can highly recommend is Bio-K, produced by Bio-K International Inc. This is a super potent Lb. acidophilus+Lb. casei. with 50 billion live active cells per serving and is 100% natural.

- Lactopriv/B is a delicious Lactobacillus that comes in powdered form.

- Natrens – Megadophilus with Bifido factor.

THE MASTER CLEANSER, OR "LEMONADE DIET"

(originated by Stanley Burroughs)

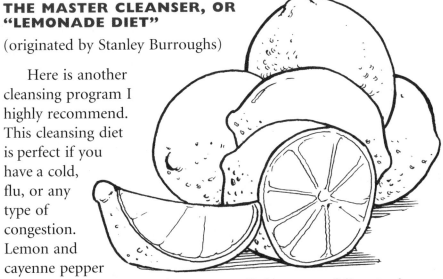

Here is another cleansing program I highly recommend. This cleansing diet is perfect if you have a cold, flu, or any type of congestion. Lemon and cayenne pepper really dislodge mucous. This program feels great to follow in the spring. I use this cleanse every year for about 10 days. I love it.

Dr. Elson Haas, author of *The Detox Diet*, also recommends this cleansing program in his book. At an I-ACT convention, Dr. Haas told us that he also does this cleanse quite often.

The creator of this program condemns the use of colonics … I love ya', Mr. Burroughs, but obviously I do not see eye-to-eye with you on this matter. I do, however, love this cleanse and don't feel that I should throw the baby out with the bath-water, if you know what I mean.

How to make it:

- 2 tablespoons lemon or lime juice (approx. ½ lemon)

- 2 tablespoons genuine maple syrup (not maple-flavored sugar syrup)

- $1/_{10}$ teaspoon cayenne pepper (red pepper) to taste

- Water (spring or purified), medium hot

Combine the juice, maple syrup, and cayenne pepper in a 10-ounce glass and fill with medium hot water (cold water may be used if preferred). Use fresh lemons or limes only, never canned lemon or lime juice, nor frozen lemonade or frozen juice. Use organic lemons whenever possible.

Purpose:

- Dissolve and eliminate toxins and congestion that have formed in any part of the body.

- Cleanse the kidneys and the digestive system.

- Purify the glands and cells throughout the entire body.

- Eliminate all unusable and hardened material in the joints and muscles.

- Relieve pressure and irritation in the nerves, arteries, and blood vessels.

- Build a healthy bloodstream.

- Keep youth and elasticity regardless of your age.

When to use it:

- When sickness has developed—for all acute and chronic conditions.

- When the digestive system needs a rest and a cleansing.

- When obesity has become a problem.

- When better assimilation and building of body tissue is needed.

How long and how often to use it:

Follow the diet for a minimum of 10 days. It may be safely followed for up to 40 days or more in extremely serious cases. This diet has all the nutrition needed during this time. Doing this 3 to 4 times a year will work wonders for keeping your body in a healthy state, and it may be undertaken more frequently for serious conditions.

NO MORE WHINING ... NO MORE EXCUSES!

I am confused . . . I don't understand these cleansing programs.

Puh-leeez! This is not brain surgery. Don't take the position of learned helplessness. With all the reference books (and for Pete's sake, let's not forget this book!) I have provided, you could be an expert in detoxification if you really wanted to. You have a pretty weak argument here. I think you just need to get off your petukis and get to it, already.

I just can't swallow all these pills!

Let me tell you the true story of a young girl about 8 years old who thought she just couldn't swallow pills. One day her mother tried to get her to take some vitamin supplements. They were in their kitchen, which was separated from the front door by a slatted wooden divider. The young girl was so resistant to swallowing the pills that a struggle ensued and she found herself backed up against the divider. Then, to her mother's horror, the little girl's head got stuck between the wooden slats. Fortunately, the mother got her daughter's head unstuck—or I would not be sitting here writing this book. Yes, I was that little girl. My mother worked with me until I was soon able to

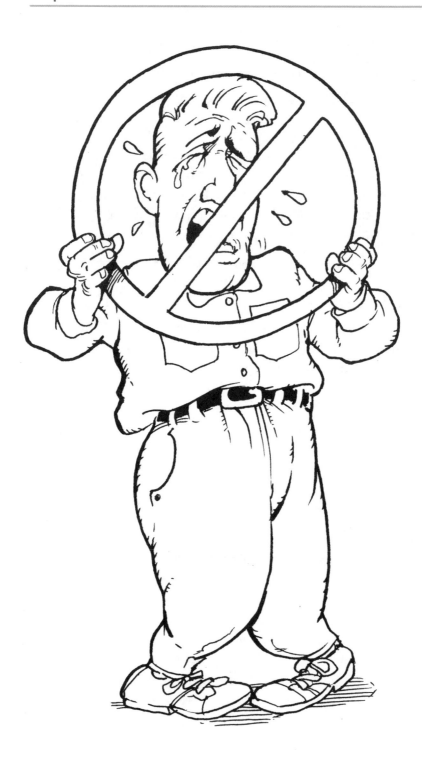

swallow several pills at a time. Resistance and fear just make the whole process harder for everybody. Talk with a cancer patient who is making every effort to save his life, and find out what he is going through—taking pills, shots, medications, and IV's. Maybe this will help put things in perspective for you.

What if I don't like the cleansing drink?

So what if you don't? Drink it anyway. This program does not have to be a big inconvenience unless you make it so. If you had a life-threatening health condition and your doctor told you that drinking this medication would save your life, I'll bet you would get creative and figure out a way to drink it. As the saying goes, "Where there's a will, there's a way."

I don't have time to detoxify.

You are right. You can wait until you are confined to bed with a life-threatening illness, maybe even cancer, if you are lucky. Cancer is really going to take a chunk out of your social life ... you will have plenty of time then.

I can't afford it!

You are right again. You can't afford any herbs or colonics. You have to start saving your money. Take another look at Chapter 9 on cancer—you had better put away at least about $50,000 to $75,000 for your cancer treatments.

I can't go without eating for 7 days.

Right again. It will probably be much easier for you to get used to it when they are feeding you intravenously.

My family thinks its weird. They won't support this endeavor!

Get a new family.

I am too embarrassed to go in for a professional colonic!

Get over it!

291

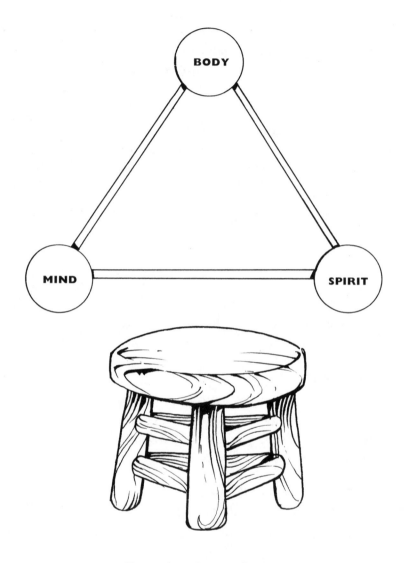

Examine Your Stool

If just one leg of a three-legged stool is shorter than the others it will tip over. We are spiritual human beings who need balance in our lives. We must have our body, mind, and spirit balanced at all times, so we, too, don't tip over.

CHAPTER 21

■ ■ ■ ■ ■ ■ ■ ■ ■ ■ ■

The Body-Mind Connection

We can detoxify, eat a perfect diet, and still not get well. Our physical health (body) is directly related to our mental and spiritual attitudes. As with a three-legged stool, if we are out of balance in any of these areas (body, mind, or spirit), our stool will tip over. I believe we tip over when we become un-balanced long enough to create a disease process. If we are mentally or spiritually bankrupt, our body will manifest this.

According to Louise Hay (author of *Heal Your Body*), the mental thought patterns that most often cause disease in the body are criticism, anger, resentment, and guilt. For instance, criticism indulged in long enough will often lead to diseases such as arthritis. Anger turns into things that boil and burn and infect the body. Long-held resentment festers and eats away at the self, and ultimately can lead to tumors and cancer. Guilt always seeks punishment and leads to pain. It is so much easier to release these negative thinking patterns from our minds when we are healthy than to try to dig them out when we are in a state of panic and under the threat of the surgeon's knife. If we are to take responsibility for our health, without blaming, and if we truly want the health God has for us, then we must change our attitudes and ourselves. No one can do this for us. We must take responsibility.

HEALING ATTITUDES

The following are healing attitudes from *Teach Only Love* by Dr. Jerry Jampolsky.

- ◆ *Health is inner peace.* Therefore, healing is in letting go of fear. If we make changing the body our goal, we fail to recognize that our single most important goal is peace of mind. The essence of your being is love. Love cannot be hindered by what is merely physical. Therefore, we believe the mind has no limits, nothing is impossible, and all disease is potentially reversible. And because love is eternal, death need not be viewed as something to fear.

- ◆ *Giving is receiving.* When our attention is on giving and joining with others, fear is removed and we accept healing for ourselves.

- ◆ *All minds are joined.* Therefore, all healing is self-healing. Our inner peace will of itself transmit to others once we accept it for ourselves.

- ◆ *Now is the only time there is.* Pain, grief, depression, guilt, and other forms of fear disappear when the mind is focused in loving peace on this instant. Decisions are made by learning to listen to the preference for peace within us. There is no completely right or wrong behavior. The only meaningful choice is between fear and love.

- ◆ *Forgiveness is the way to true health and happiness.* By not judging, we release the past and let go of our fears of the future. In so doing, we come to see that everyone is our teacher and that every circumstance is an opportunity for growth in happiness, peace and love.

HEALING OUR RELATIONSHIPS, HEALING OURSELVES

In his book, *Think and Be Healthy,* Jim Jenks gives us three attitudes to help heal our relationships:

◆ *Appreciation.* Show appreciation. By seeking mentally the positive traits of others, you will automatically start showing appreciation. Do you like to be appreciated? Well then, be generous with appreciation.

◆ *Forgiveness.* In the name of health, forgive. Give yourself permission to make a mistake as you would give permission to your spouse, child, or friend. Forgive daily. Forgiveness is the key to and basis of your healing attitude.

◆ *Feeling needed.* To feel needed is a strong basic human requirement. Let your family and friends know that you need them. Be sincere.

HONOR YOUR HEART AND YOUR EMOTIONS

I like to ask: "Who are you?" I know your name, what you look like, but really deep down in your core, in your heart and soul, who are you? What do you value? What are your dreams? Have you lived your whole life being someone that your parents, spouse, and friends wanted you to be, or are you being who you want yourself to be?

Are you in touch with your true authentic self? Do you speak up and say what you mean and mean what you say? Do you stand up for your values and your core beliefs, or do you sell yourself out so that you won't make waves or go against the grain? Do you do things in your daily life that nurture and feed your soul? If you are not feeding your body physically, mentally, and spiritually, you will feel unbalanced and tip over your stool.

Real Moments

by Loree Taylor Jordan

Thank your creator every day.
Dance like no one is watching.
Give people more than they expect.
Laughter is healing ... laugh 'til it hurts.
Be generous to yourself and others.
Work like you don't need the money.
Really listen to people with an open heart.
Say I am sorry ... first!
Run with scissors—take risks.
Remember, life is a gift ... love your life.
Sing like no one is listening.
Goof off, laugh at yourself, and play every day.
Love like you've never been hurt.
Be outrageous and silly ...
Don't take yourself so seriously.
Honor your wisdom and trust your heart.
Show love and courage ...
Positively impact others.
Say "I love you" ... first!
Be grateful and show appreciation.
Be forgiving of yourself and others.
Be open to possibility ...
Speak from your heart.
Always speak your truth.
Look in the mirror at the most beautiful
smile in the world ... yours!

I extend to you all
my friendship, love, and support.

*Feel free to copy these affirmations and
pass them on to others with my blessing.*

IT IS TIME TO STEP UP

It's up to you and you alone to step up to a higher standard. No more "I don't know," learned helplessness, or convenient excuses; no more procrastination. Release yourself from negative attitudes. Pray to God and ask Him to take away your unwanted and unhealthy attitudes and character defects, and to restructure you with positive, healthy attitudes. Be forgiving of yourself and others. Be humble in your heart and your spirit. Remember: *Nothing changes until something changes.*

HEALING AFFIRMATIONS

I am a loving person, created in God's image.

I am vibrant and alive and I radiate health to everyone.

With the help of God, I am invincible, invulnerable, and unshakable.

Whatever happens, I remain calm ... composed ... self-confident.

I can face reality ... and I am able to meet any life situation.

I am indifferent to any emotional stress and disappointment.

Regardless of contrary negative thoughts, I am able to act positively.

God gives me abundant life and health ... I am well and beautiful.

I maintain an attitude of gratitude.

> *He who has health has hope,*
> *and he who has hope has everything.*
> – Arab proverb

CHAPTER 22

■ ■ ■ ■ ■ ■ ■ ■ ■ ■ ■

The Cleansing Power of Water

*In health and in sickness, pure water is one of
the choicest blessings. It is the beverage given by
God to quench the thirst of man and animal,
and to cleanse the poisons from our system.*

— Byrne

I cannot overemphasize the importance of super-hydrating your body with liberal amounts of water on a daily basis. Water is the largest single component of the human body. It is stated that our brains are said to be 85% water. Water is the essence of life. Blood, digestive juices, perspiration, tears; the list of water-based solutions that make our bodies function goes on and on. Every bodily function is monitored and designed around the efficient intake and flow of water. This water distribution is the only way of making sure its transported elements such as hormones, oxygen, and nutrients reach our vital organs. We depend on water to hydrate our cells. We absolutely cannot survive without water.

F. Batmanghelidj, M.D. in his book *Your Body's Many Cries for Water* states, "One of the unavoidable processes in the body's water rationing phase is the complete cruelty with which some functions are monitored so that one structure does not receive more that its predetermined share of water. This is true for all organs of the body. Within these systems of water rationing, the brain function takes absolute priority over all the other systems — the brain is $1/50^{th}$ of the total body weight, but it receives 18 to 20 percent of blood circulation. When the 'ration masters' in charge of regulating and distributing the body water reserve become more and more active, they also give their own alarm signals to show that the area in question is short of water, very much like the radiator of a car gives out steam when the cooling system is not adequate for an uphill drive."

The success of any cleansing program is only as successful as your commitment to take in adequate amounts of water. It is suggested you divide your body weight by 2, and consume this many ounces of water every day (for example, if you weigh 120 pounds, drink 60 ounces of water). During any cleansing program I suggest about a gallon of water every day. Water is the cornerstone for detoxifying all the organs and cells of the body. By drinking liberal amounts of water we reduce the acid buildup that has been stored in various organs such as the heart, liver, colon, as well as connective tissue and joints. Let us take this one step further and say that this over-acid condition is a degenerative disease and the aging process in the making.

When I consult with my clients I cannot believe how many people think that fluid and water are synonymous. Water is water, anything else is not. I am talking pure water not coffee, tea, sodas and all the sugar-laden, manufactured beverages that unfortunately serve as substitutes for water. It is true that these beverages contain water, but they also contain dehydrating agents. Dehydrating agents, such as those in coffee and sodas, deplete the body of its water reserves.

Children are the worst victims of nutritionally uneducated parents. They are brought up at a young age on manufactured juices and soda drinks and they become addicted. More than once I have seen — I am telling you the absolute truth here —

young toddlers with soda pop in their baby bottles. I had not completely embarked on my nutritional path at that point in my life or God knows what I would have said to those parents. *Soda in a baby bottle?!* Don't get me started.

Now, to add insult to injury, one of the main components of most sodas is caffeine, an addictive drug. If you don't think so, just go cold turkey from coffee or caffeine sodas and you will get a migraine headache you will never forget. I used to be a diet Pepsi addict. When I started my cleanse (many, many years ago) for three long days I thought the top of my head would explode! There are soda pop junkies who are addicts just like alcoholics, drug addicts, and cigarette smokers. Drinking soda is more socially acceptable, but just as deadly.

Dr. Batmanghelidj, MD goes on to say that "Caffeine's addictive properties are due to its direct action in the brain. It also acts on the kidneys and causes increased urine production. Caffeine has diuretic properties. It is physiologically a dehydrating agent. This prime characteristic is the main reason a person is forced to drink so many cans of soda every day and never be satisfied. The water does not stay in the body long enough. At the same time, many persons confuse their feeling of thirst for water; thinking they have consumed enough 'water' in the soda, they assume they are hungry and begin to eat more than their body's need for food."

Along with caffeine, sugar, and aspartame (sweetener in diet sodas), we must also consider the effects of phosphoric acid. According to John Thomas, author of *Young Again,* "The side effects of soft drinks loaded with phosphoric acid are incomprehensible and go beyond just our pH level. When ingested, the body is forced to draw on bone calcium to buffer the acid introduced into the bloodstream, which skews the calcium phosphorous ration and grossly alters body physiology. When the side effects of aspartame sweetener are added, it's a wonder we don't just die!"

Okay, you say, you are convinced now that chronic cellular dehydration is detrimental to your overall health. You agree that drinking adequate water is a not a *should* but a *must* for optimal health! Another question to consider: Is all water equal in its benefits to the body? Just as with food, you could choose a greasy hamburger or a fresh salad. Both are considered food but do they have the same benefit to the body? A hamburger is a *devitalized dead* food devoid of enzymes; a salad is fresh *live* food with enzymes intact. The body would utilize and break down these two foods differently. So it is with water. Water can come in two forms: live water or dead water.

I could recite a lot of scientific mumbo jumbo but let's just keep this simple and to the point. The goal in drinking water is to get that water to the cellular level for energy and to hydrate the cells rapidly. If the water is not able to get deep down into the cells themselves, then the body will not completely benefit from it. Let's consider how water that is molecularly restructured can handle this issue. We will see that all water is not created equal.

In considering a water source we want a water that is molecularly superior for our optimal health. One water that I use and can recommend is Penta-Hydrate™, produced by Bio-Hydration Research Lab located in San Diego, California. The "3G" of water—it is the third generation of performance-enhancing water after bottled water and "oxygenated water"—Penta Hydrate™ energizes the body faster by hydrating cells rapidly. The following is taken from their product report which I requested to pass on to you, my readers.

Bio-Hydration Laboratory, in an experiment to remove dissolved solids from water, discovered their test water maintained its clustered molecular state which, under normal circumstances only happens for a short, unsustainable period of time. In the human body, H_2o resides in one of two molecular states: bound and clustered.

Bound water is attached to other molecules, ions and free radicals, making it thicker and prohibiting it from moving through cell walls via osmosis. In other words, bound water simply cannot hydrate cells. Unfortunately for the water drinker, water exists in this bound state 85% of the time.

The importance of this discovery is paramount because water in its clustered state is another story. Clustered water passes through cell walls effortlessly because it's smaller, unbound from the molecules that weigh down bound water. But due to water's complexities and instability, clustered water only exists for short periods of time and in very small amounts. At any given moment, only 15% of the water we are drinking is in this clustered state.

So, simply put (I like to keep things simple ... chemistry is not my forté), water can only penetrate the cells in a clustered state. So a live water such as Penta-Hydrate™ that is molecularly restructured to stay in this clustered state solves this problem. I was introduced to Penta-Hydrate™ water at Life Mastery with Tony Robbins and noticed a very different taste immediately. It is very smooth ... I personally love it.

MEDICAL GRADE IONIZED WATER™

In his book *Young Again*, John Thomas explains about a special class of therapeutic water used in special Japanese clinics to treat everything from diabetes and nerve disorders to cancer and heart/stroke problems. In his book Mr. Thomas describes this process.

In Japan, this special water is made with very expensive equipment designed for clinical settings. In the USA, where tap water pollutant levels are gross, the BEV™ process is used to create "conception point" water with a biologically friendly ORP (oxidized-reduction-potential) and a "clear" memory.

Medical Grade Ionized Water™ *is then made from BEV™ water and racemized™ with liquid minerals. Raw tap water is* never *used. It is vitally important that the reader understand that the pH (acid/alkalinity) of this special water is* not *what does the healing. Rather, it is the ORP potential which is a measurement of electron availability for mitochondrial production of the energy molecule, ATP.*

The benefits of high ORP water derive from a combination of purity, ORP, resistivity, and pH. Highly reduced *acid water and highly* oxidized *alkaline water have pH values of 1.5 to 2.4 and 10.5 to 12, respectively, and ORP potentials of −900 and +1200 respectively. High ORP water is composed of tiny water molecules that easily cross cell membranes so the reduced water can deliver its load of electrons to the mitochondria for increased ATP production and tissue rejuvenation. Disease has its roots at the cellular level, which is where high ORP Medical Grade Water™ does its job.*

Oxidized *water is used externally to heal infections, for douches, in treatment of genital herpes, and for beautiful skin. Reduced water is taken orally at the rate of ¾ to 1 gallon a day, thereby pumping the body with energy while neutralizing acid wastes, similar to the way a Far InfraRed™ sauna deacidifies the soft tissues without the use of heat, steam or lights. Medical Grade Ionized Water™ is one of the biggest health advances in medical history.*

Many times I have been asked about drinking tap water. Drinking tap water is slow suicide at best. I'd hoped that common sense would absolve me from even having to mention it here, but then again, remember soda pop in a toddler's bottle? Where was common sense in that scenario? Let's cut to the chase and get straight to the point. Tap water is a Pandora's box

> *We are now at the dawn of a new era in medical science. It is chronic water shortage in the body that causes most of the disease of the human body. The original design of the human body is more complete than you can imagine. If we have not known how to maintain it until now, it is our own fault. We have not stopped to think, if the body is mainly water, where will it get its top-up if we don't drink water on a regular basis? We now know when it is calling for its urgent intake. We need to dwell on this information. Pushing water is not a personal gimmick. There is no hidden agenda to its promotion—if you share this information with your loved ones, you are its beneficiary.*
>
> – F. Batmanghelidi, MD
> *Your Body's Many Cries For Water*

of bacteria, chemical pollutants, toxins, carcinogens, etc., etc. Tap water? ... don't even go there. Never consider drinking it! End of story!

I receive no financial gain whatsoever from either one of these companies. I just want to be a resource for you to receive your God-given right to optimal health. Information for both of these companies is in the Resource Guide, so you may contact them for ordering or additional product information.

FINAL THOUGHTS

I know that I have used a lot of humor in this book, but please understand that, with ultimate seriousness and respect, I am dedicated to detoxification and cleansing of the human body. You would not even consider going weeks without a shower (or at least I hope you wouldn't), or months without washing your hair, so why would the inside of your body be any less important?

Really, if you don't have a healthy body, where are you going to live? What do you value in your life? Your health ... your time ... your family? Which is it? Life is so precious and fragile. Please do not take it for granted. Life and health can be jerked away from any of us at any given moment. When health is lost we will pay anything to get well, to save our life or that of our loved one. Think of how your priorities would change if you found out tomorrow that you or a loved one had a life-threatening illness that could have been prevented. I implore you to think of detoxification as prevention ... the best health insurance you can buy.

Please do not be overwhelmed by all the valuable information provided in this book. You must take one step at a time ... but take the step! You may just start with proper food combining then find a colon therapist in your area. You might dive in head first and call a local colon therapist, tell them you just read my book—you want to cleanse your body no matter how long it takes!

You may become a colon evangelist and pass my book to family and friends. Who knows what your reaction will be, but from the bottom of my heart and soul I implore you to do something proactive to cleanse and detoxify your body for vital health. You and only you have full control to a positive and healthy outcome. No passing the buck here!

Health is your wealth. Guard it with knowledge, then put your knowledge into action. If I have given you new tools to take good care of your body, I am grateful. In the process, if I have made you laugh, I am truly blessed.

Remember ... always examine your stool!

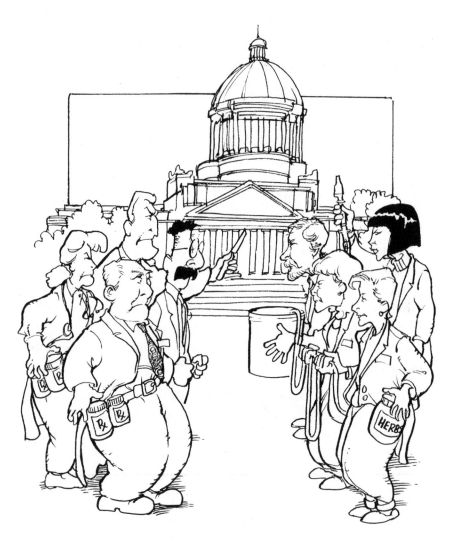

Shootout at the OK Corral

CHAPTER 23

■ ■ ■ ■ ■ ■ ■ ■ ■ ■

Politics & Science

All truth passes through three stages: first it is ridiculed; second, it is violently opposed; third, it is accepted as being self-evident.

– Schoepenhauer

THE COLON HYDROTHERAPY CONTROVERSY

Segments of the medical community discriminate against colon hydrotherapy, despite its centuries-old record of benefits to patients. For example, some doctors have objected to colon hydrotherapy on the grounds that it is an invasive procedure. With that logic, however, teeth brushing and douching the vaginal area are invasive procedures. Is the insertion of a foreign object into an opening of the body as invasive a procedure as surgery?

There have been changes in my own practice in the administration of the speculum (the tube that is inserted into the rectum) into the client. At one point as a colon hydrotherapist I was allowed—in my scope of practice—to perform a digital exam with a gloved hand (with permission of the client). The reason for the digital exam was to make an assessment of the quality of the sphincter muscles before insertion of the speculum. It was often appropriate to dilate the sphincter muscles to relax the client for easier insertion. Then I was informed by IACT (International Association of Colon Hydrotherapy) that we could no longer perform a digital exam because the medical community considered it an invasive procedure. We were told instead to have the clients insert the speculum into the rectum themselves, so we would not be accused of performing an invasive procedure.

Many of my clients objected to doing it themselves, stating to me, "Look, I am a consenting adult and if I consent to having a speculum inserted into my rectum by you as my colon hydrotherapist then I have that right to decide." This discrimination and ignorance from the medical community was taken all the way to the Senate in July 1992.

ASSEMBLY BILL AB 856

The following section is excerpted from *Stay Young and Healthy Through Internal Cleansing* by Millan Chessman. She has graciously given me permission to share her research and data regarding the Senate Bill AB 856.

◆ ◆ ◆

The following is an example of misinformation. In December of 1991, Ken Douglas of the Medical Board of California received this letter from a former president of the California Medical Association, Laurens P. White, MD, Internal Medicine and Oncology, of San Francisco:

Dear Mr. Douglas:

I am writing [to state] that the performance of colonic irrigation, a practice clearly condemned by the medical and chiropractic professions, is very much an element of the practice of medicine that is outlawed. I know of no reputable physician or chiropractor who performs this procedure any longer.

Colonic irrigation (or flushing) has been outlawed for several good reasons. These are:

1. It has no useful therapeutic functions.

2. Whether done with water, coffee, or liquids, it is without benefit.

3. It is dangerous, and may result in rupture of the bowel, peritonitis, or unusual fluid absorption.

For these reasons no one should perform this disreputable pseudo-therapy, and anyone performing it should be considered guilty of unprofessional conduct.

Yours truly,
Laurens P. White, MD

As you can see this letter is filled with false statements. This doctor probably had never known any recipient of colon hydrotherapy or any colon hydrotherapist. Assemblywoman Tricia Hunter, who had once been a nurse, snatched up this letter. She apparently saw it as an opportunity to produce legislation in the California State Assembly, and introduced Assembly Bill 856. As if by way of endorsement of her actions, the California Medical Association was the largest contributor to Hunter's re-election campaign, chipping in with a whopping $12,500. Leslie Williams noted the following in a response to Hunter's AB 856: "The files of the California Secretary of State, March Fong Eu, [revealed that] Tricia Hunter received a check for $5,000 from the CMA on April 8, 1992, the day before the bill was introduced and a second check for $7,500 ... a month later, on May 9, 1992."

Except as it pertains to chiropractors, there is, in fact, no California law against obtaining or administering colon hydrotherapy. The therapy is not "an element of the practice of medicine which has been outlawed." If "no reputable physicians or chiropractors ... perform this procedure any longer," then why the necessity for a law? There are no reported cases of ruptured bowels, peritonitis, or unusual fluid absorption due to colon hydrotherapy in over 150 years anywhere in the United States! There are, however, such cases due to improperly administered enemas.

> *Fact: Since colon hydrotherapy became a "profession" in the middle of the 19th century in North America, there have been no reports of injuries. The one case cited by AB 856 in Colorado was amoeba contamination.*

The one incident that has been cited as a reason to outlaw colon hydrotherapy occurred over 25 years ago. It had nothing to do with the therapy or the technique of administration. It did involve a tank and reusable hose that was joined together outside the body. Unfortunately, the person using the equipment did not bother to change the hoses between sessions, allowing the next client to be infected with the previous client's contaminants. After a client suffering from amoebic dysentery came in for several sessions, 33 people were infected through the unsanitary hoses.

Leslie Williams, President of the International Association for Colon Hydrotherapists, states the following:

> *No one died after getting colon hydrotherapy. Those who died did so after bowel surgery performed by the medical doctors. The session itself did not cause any illness. It was the unsanitary conditions where the patients contracted amoebas.*

Gregory Istre, MD, wrote an article in the *New England Journal of Medicine* on the spread of amoebiasis via colon hydrotherapy. Leslie Williams interviewed him. He told her he was "surprised that the California Medical Association used this article to try to outlaw a whole profession."

Assemblywoman Tricia Hunter, from the Palm Springs area, carried this legislation. It was introduced April 9, 1992, in the middle of the second half of the 2-year legislative term.

Within a week of the bill being discovered, the legislators' offices in the capital in Sacramento, California, resounded with phone calls, letters, and personal visits. The unfortunate assemblyman who had co-authored the bill (before it was gutted and replaced with the new legislation) hurriedly removed his name from the bill.

He had no knowledge that the bill had been changed. The number of indignant people calling to demand that the piece be dropped overwhelmed his clerical staff. The assemblyman's staff felt they should be answering the phone: "Colon Hydrotherapy Central."

One of the staff members of a senator on the health committee marveled that of the thousands of bills introduced each legislative session, none had created the furor that this one had, other than one concerning water rights due to the drought. The bill had one hearing and was tabled due to lack of documented proof of causing harm.

In 1984, John Luly, a chiropractor in San Diego, advertised colon hydrotherapy as a cure for various ailments. The California Medical Board sued him and, after years in court, the judge ruled against the chiropractor. Chiropractors could no longer administer colon hydrotherapy although colon hydrotherapy had been part of the chiropractor's scope of practice in California. At that, the Chiropractic Examining Board sued the California Medical Association to establish that chiropractors could indeed perform colon hydrotherapy. This was paid for out of public funds allocated by the Attorney General. This suit lasted seven years and cost $2 million of taxpayers' money. Cause and effect of colon hydrotherapy were not at issue. It was simply a turf war. The end result was that the chiropractors were going to lose, so they dropped the suit and agreed to back legislation outlawing the procedure as a concession to pressure from the California Medical Association.

The California Medical Association wrote the proposed assembly bill thinking, no doubt, it had a no-contest case, and that the bill would pass without anyone's awareness, since the general populace is fairly uninformed about the benefits of colon hydrotherapy (as are most member doctors in the CMA).

AB 856 Controversy Continues

For a field as obscure as colon hydrotherapy, the outcry was loud. Only two interests supported AB 856: the CMA (California Medical Association) and California's Board of Chiropractic Examiners. This second group had lost countless members in a mass exodus from its rolls, and 256 individuals went on record with letters of protest to the California State Senate Health and Human Services Committee.

The groups opposed to AB 856 were:

- ◆ American Colon Therapist Association
- ◆ California Colon Therapy Society
- ◆ Specialty Health Products
- ◆ Laguna Medical Center, Inc.
- ◆ Wellness Associates
- ◆ Dotolo Research Corporation
- ◆ Church of Golden Light
- ◆ California Nurses Association
- ◆ California Chiropractic Association

MD's Speak Out for Colon Hydrotherapy

Medical doctors were among those individuals who cared enough to take the time to write to their state representatives. Ron Kennedy, an MD from Rohnert Park, California, wrote a letter to Senate Health and Human Services Committee Chairperson, Diane Watson, explaining that he had studied colon hydrotherapy for two years and had concluded:

It is a valuable procedure which, in trained hands, is as safe as any procedure performed on the human body can be.

Dr. Kennedy stated that he also considered it "extremely useful as a method of preventing serious colon disease." He recommended that if any regulatory action were taken, it be along the lines of Florida policy, which licenses colon hydrotherapy as an adjunct to massage therapy. Kennedy pointed out that medical schools provide no training in colon hydrotherapy, and that medical physicians are "trained to handle the body after disease is present and perhaps even life-threatening." He went on to make the remarkable statement, considering he is a medical doctor: that physicians "have little interest, as a group, in prevention of illness."

In another paper, Kennedy writes:

In my view it would be unconstitutional to outlaw the practice of colonics by colon therapists and leave it to medical doctors who know next to nothing about the prevention of colon disease. Most colon therapists are convinced, as I certainly am, that the great increase in colon cancer over the past few generations is also due to autointoxication in the colon. High-fiber foods change the bacterial flora of your colon to non-carcinogenic organisms and drastically reduce the possibility of colon cancer. Medical doctors are not trained to deal with the colon until it becomes severely diseased.

In his work, Dr. Kennedy concludes that putrefying waste material causes autointoxication and leads to dangerous pre-cancerous conditions in the colon. In addition, various other gastrointestinal complaints and diseases are associated with a poisoned bowel. Kennedy connects the effects of toxicity with other ailments seemingly unrelated to the bowel. In his view, medical doctors of all specialties find it difficult to treat these problems successfully due to their ignorance of a sick bowel as a possible root cause of illness.

Another opponent of AB 856, John W. Travis, MD, MPH, of Sebastopol, California, wrote the following to Chairperson Watson:

> I'm shocked at the apparent attempt to outlaw colon hydrotherapy via AB 856. While I do not practice it myself, I believe it is one of many important forms of treatment that we were not taught in medical school ... I hope you and your committee will provide the much-needed leadership to prevent such regressive legislation from occurring.

In agreement, Bessie Jo Tillman, MD, of Redding, also wrote to the committee:

> I frequently refer [constipated] patients for colon [hydro]therapy ... I have never had problems with serious injuries or illnesses, such as infection, bowel perforation, bowel necrosis [death of the bowel tissues caused by use of caustic soaps or other irritants that attack the delicate lining of the colon] ... With the sophisticated and refined temperatures and pressure gauges, disposable tubing and speculum, and trained, certified hydrotherapists ... I have only obtained positive results. I have never had complaints.

Elson M. Haas, MD, and director of a clinic in San Rafael, states that in over 15 years of referring hundreds of patients to colon hydrotherapists for treatment, he has "never seen any medical complications." He goes on to explain the safety and efficacy of modern internal cleansing practices, and ultimately says: "There is essentially no risk of medical problem. The statements in the current Assembly Bill 856 about the hazards of colon [hydrotherapy] are simply erroneous. This simple procedure cannot cause bowel necrosis and death, and in well-trained hands with proper techniques there is no risk of infection and bowel perforation."

Paul Lynn, MD, of San Francisco, had this to say to the Senate Health and Human Services Committee:

> *I feel that this form of natural health care is falsely represented and that the information in the upcoming Assembly Bill 856 regarding these procedures, claiming they are harmful and dangerous, is totally inaccurate. I have often referred patients to get [colon hydrotherapy] from a qualified therapist [who] uses proven, sophisticated equipment, including a refined pressure gauge along with disposable tubing. I have received only positive reports from these sessions and if it were not safe and sanitary, I would not recommend them. I urge you to reconsider this unconstitutional bill from being passed into law.*

This sampling shows the outcry from an informed segment of the medical community. A number of celebrities were unafraid to make a public stand for the practice of colon hydrotherapy. In fact, many movie stars who regularly receive colon hydrotherapy submitted letters to senators and assembly-people protesting the passage of AB 856.

A Biased Doctor Responds

At the other end of the spectrum, the CMA's Frederick H. Noteware, Assistant Director of Government Relations, wrote in support of AB 856 to the CMA's "expert" witness, President Richard F. Corlin, MD:

> *I am taking this opportunity to pass along to you comments I have received from those who advocate the administration of colonic irrigation:*
>
> *1. From Nancy McBride, chiropractor: "If a person needs an enema, they certainly need a colonic irrigation."*
>
> *"Why?"*
>
> *"Because the body gets toxic."*

"What does that mean?"

"There's feedback into the liver."

2. There are people who consider themselves to be "colon therapists" after having received training and certification at some as yet unnamed institution. I'm beginning to hear what they may suggest as a compromise: ... amend AB 856 (Hunter) to create a new category of licensure for colon therapists. I have explained this would be absolutely unacceptable for a variety of reasons, not the least of which is the fact the administration of a colonic irrigation is an invasive procedure, and under the law (with few exceptions), only physicians are affected. My view is if the "colon therapists" offer licensure as a compromise, it supports our position since they are acknowledging the inherent value in protecting the public health from untrained practitioners.

3. When asked why colonics are necessary, the common response is usually "to remove the toxins."

4. When pressed as to the therapeutic value, the answer is "Well, they make you feel better." I always follow that answer with the question, "Can you provide me with any documented, peer-reviewed, scientific literature to suggest any medical reason to drain the colon?" The answer is always no.

5. Other comments:

    a. "Physicians do not receive any nutritional training so they wouldn't know the benefits of colon therapy."

    b. "Wheatgrass enemas have been especially helpful with cancer patients."

    c. "This is a freedom of choice issue with my body."

*d. "This bill is self-serving by the CMA and
motivated by money interests."*

The arrogance and laziness of AB 856's supporters within the CMA became apparent with this cynical letter by Noteware. There is no attempt to dig deeper than the surface. Noteware might not have written such a frivolous and contemptuous recommendation if he had had an open mind, and had performed an unbiased review of the literature, contacted any colon hydrotherapy association, used up some shoe leather to personally interview and observe both practitioners and their clients, or talked to the doctors who prescribe the procedure. But the gilded status accorded to the mere fact of a medical degree in anything—however strong or weak the actual qualifying marks to receive it—seems to have blinded Mr. Noteware to his own erroneous assumptions.

Dr. Corlin, evidently busy as he was, did not subsequently take the time, either, to find out the facts about colon hydrotherapy before he was scheduled to testify to the HHS Committee. Inexplicably, he neglected to clarify to himself the difference between an enema and colon hydrotherapy. The transcript of the hearing itself is a testimony to arrogant ignorance. Neither Hunter nor Corlin were able to present a satisfactory case for AB 856, and only succeeded in frustrating and wearying the Committee by refusing to differentiate between enemas and colon hydrotherapy.

Members of the committee asked for substantiation that the therapy is dangerous, ineffective, or useless. Interestingly, Corlin could not provide it. Members of the Committee made reference to the mail they had received on this issue, and even admitted to some personal knowledge of the procedure and its beneficial outcome. One Committee member, Senator Mello, used the example of tonsillectomy to illustrate that he was not convinced the medical establishment automatically and infallibly knows everything at any time about any aspect of health.

Corlin and company were not pleased by these disclosures. They left with their tails between their legs.

The Death of AB 856

The upshot of the hearing was the defeat of Hunter's bill. As chairperson Senator Watson stated, AB 856 was full of "loopholes big enough to drive a Mack truck through." She advised Assemblywoman Hunter to take the bill back to the drawing board, and if merited, to present it again another time.

AB 856 was not passed that July 1992. Since that time, CMA has not been in communication with the IACT, nor has it pursued any efforts to outlaw colon hydrotherapy.

– *Stay Young and Healthy Through Internal Cleansing*
by Millan Chessman

◆ ◆ ◆

(I want to thank Millan Chessman for sharing her research with all of us. This information is a huge contribution to this book and I am grateful.)

MY TWO CENTS

I was at that Senate meeting in Sacramento in 1992 when medical doctors were trying to sneak through AB 856 outlawing colon hydrotherapy, saying colonics had absolutely no medical value. This meeting was what my father would call a "three-ring circus." I have to say that it was a huge display of ignorance on the part of the medical doctors present. They continued to insist that colon hydrotherapists were just trying to rip people off and our services provided no documented value whatsoever.

They even went as far as to say that people had died from colon hydrotherapy. Senator Henry Mello was great. He asked these doctors to produce proof of any deaths from colonic treatment. Of course these doctors could not produce any proof, nor bereaved family members of these supposed colonic fatalities. Do you know why? *Because there weren't any!* You can see from Millan's research that deaths were from bowel surgery, not colon hydrotherapy. It's like saying you shouldn't brush your teeth to remove the plaque—it might be too dangerous.

I am sorry that the doctors present at this Senate meeting did not educate themselves before presenting their inaccurate claims to the Senate Committee. They should at least have interviewed some of the members of the medical community who support colon hydrotherapy.

Eight years after this fiasco the public is still being warned by well-meaning (but ignorant) doctors about the physical and financial dangers of colon hydrotherapy. Just recently I read several articles published in major magazines (*Glamour* and *Cosmopolitan*) showing this same biased ignorance of colon hydrotherapy. I've seen it mentioned that colon hydrotherapists are "hosing" the public. There has been a committee formed (of colon hydrotherapists) to present a rebuttal article to these major magazines.

In Chapter 12 of this book there is tremendous validation from MDs in support of colon hydrotherapy and detoxification. There are many physicians with many differing viewpoints. Please find one that supports your goals and viewpoint.

All I can say is I would love to send one of these doctors a jar full of the black plaque from someone's intestines and ask them if we are all imagining this "stuff." I would love to have them explain to me what this material is and why it smells like a decaying corpse.

> *Let us first understand the facts,*
> *and then we may seek the cause.*
>
> – Aristotle

CHAPTER 24

∎ ∎ ∎ ∎ ∎ ∎ ∎ ∎ ∎ ∎

Resource Guide

Alternative Cancer Treatment Information

Alternative Cancer Therapies   (323) 663-7801
The Cancer Control Society   www.cancercontrolsociety.com
2043 N. Berendo St.
Los Angeles, CA 90027

*Information available to members: Cancer Control Journal, clinic
directory, patient list, books, tapes, conventions, and clinic tours.
There is hope! Many people have found several possible approaches
to the cancer problem, such as nontoxic therapies including laetril,
gerson, hoxsey, koch, enzymes, immunology, wheatgrass, mega-
vitamins, and minerals all currently suppressed in this country.
The Cancer Control Society is a nonprofit, tax-exempt educational
society supported by memberships and donations. (Please do not
confuse this organization with the American Cancer Society.)*

National Health Federation   (626) 357-2181
P.O. Box 688
Monrovia, CA 91017

*Founded in 1955, the NHF is a nonprofit consumer education
and health organization. For 44 years they have lobbied in
Washington and state capitols to protect your right to alternative
health care, and to buy vitamins, minerals, enzymes, amino acids,
and herbs without a prescription. They provide cutting-edge information on alternative healing through magazines, newsletters,*

talks, and exhibits at health shows; and have funded lawsuits to protect the rights of alternative doctors, chiropractors, and health food store owners. You can receive their magazine, The Health Freedom News.

Alternative Practitioners & Physicians

Arthur Brawer, MD   (732) 870-3133
170 Morris Ave., Suite B
Long Branch, NJ 07740

Practice limited to rheumatology. Director of Monmouth Medical Center.

Elson Haas, MD   (415) 472-2343
25 Mitchell Blvd., #8   fax (415) 472-7636
San Rafael, CA 94903   www.elsonhaas.com

Founder and director, Preventive Medical Center of Marin; and author of seven books including The NEW! False Fat Diet, The Staying Healthy Shopper's Guide, *and* Vitamins for Dummies.

Books and Alternative Health Information

American Natural Hygiene Society   www.anhs.org
P.O. Box 30630
Tampa, FL 33630

For books on diet and nutrition. Call for their health magazine subscription.

Healthy Healing Publications   www.healthyhealing.com
Linda Page
P.O. Box 436
Carmel Valley, CA 93924

Madison Publishing
P.O. Box 231
Campbell, CA 95009

orders (800) 247-6553
www.Detoxforlife.net
www.fatandfurious.net
order@bookmaster.com

Publisher of health books, tapes, CD's, Detox for Life: Your Bottom Line: It's Your Colon or Your Life *and* Fat and Furious: Overcome Your Body's Resistance to Weight Loss Now! *by Loree Taylor Jordan, CCH, ID*

New Atlantean Books
P.O. Box 9638
Santa Fe, NM 87504

(505) 983-1856
www.thinktwice.com

An excellent resource for all subjects related to children's health. They have a comprehensive website regarding the danger of vaccinations and benefits of holistic health care for children.

Vigil Ventures
2633 Windmill View
El Cajon, CA 92020

(800) 311-8222

To order Stay Young and Healthy Through Internal Cleansing *by Millan Chessman. Millan also offers supervised 7-day cleanses at her home. Call for information.*

Young Again by John Thomas
P.O. Box 1240
Mead, WA 99021-1240

(509) 465-4154
(800) 659-1882

Order John Thomas's book, Young Again, *and you will receive information to order his "Source Packet" for the water video and water book on the EBV.*

Colon Hydrotherapist Referrals

The International Association (210) 366-2888
of Colon Hydrotherapy fax (210) 366-2999
P.O. Box 461285 www.i-act.org
San Antonio, TX 78246-1285 e-mail: IACT

Specialty Health Products (800) 343-4950
21636 N. 14th Ave. #A-1 (602) 582-4950
Phoenix, AZ 85027

For a referral to a colon hydrotherapist in your area.

Health Retreats & Spas for Cleansing

Optimum Health Institute (619) 464-3346
of San Diego (800) 993-4325
6970 Central Ave. www.optimumhealth.org
Lemon Grove, CA 91945

They offer week-long programs that include the use of wheatgrass juice, enemas, colonics, massage, nutritional classes. (You may not bring your own herbs or supplements to their location.)

We Care Health Retreat (800) 888-2523
18000 Long Canyon Rd. www.wecarespa.com
Desert Hot Springs, CA 92241

Participate in a week-long fast and colon cleanse at this 13-room retreat center with a pool. They also offer colonics and massage.

Iridology

Bernard International (760) 749-2727
24360 Old Wagon Road fax (760) 749-1248
Escondido, CA 92027

For iridology information, book, tapes, and products.

International Iridology Practitioners Association
P.O. Box 3334   (888) 682-2208
Escondido, CA USA   www.iridologyassin.org

Products

Awareness Corporation   orders (800)692- 9273
25 S. Arizona Place   fax (800) 772-7112
Fifth Floor, Suite 500   sponsor ID #1090501
Chandler, AZ 85225   www.awarecorp.com

For ordering the Clear™ cleanse. Give the sponsor number to order directly. You may view product information or you can order directly from our website: www.Detoxforlife.net.

Colema Boards™
P.O. Box 34710
North Kansas, MO

You can view different examples and order colema boards at www.Detoxforlife.net.

Enema Equipment   (800) MED-LINE
Medline Industries   (800) 633-5463
One Medline Place   www.medline.com
Mundelein, IL 60060

To order the enema set-bucket type with Dynaclamp, 54 ft. tubing with Dynaclamp 22 ft. (item #DYND70104H).

Nature's Sunshine Products
P.O. Box 19005
Spanish Fork, UT

orders (800) 453-1422
www.naturessunshine.com
sponsor ID #118691-2

You can order Loree's Kick-Butt Bowel Blaster & 7-day Boot Camp Cleanse, pH testing kits, retail directly from our website: www.Detoxforlife.net. This website will also give you instructions to order directly from Nature's Sunshine at wholesale prices if you choose. You must give product stock numbers from our website and the sponsor number to order directly.

Penta-Hydrate™
Bio-Hydration
Research Lab, Inc.
6370 Nancy Ridge Drive #104
San Diego, CA 92121

(858) 452-8868
(800) 531-5088
www.hydrateforlife.com

Penta-Hydrate™ water is available in some health food stores or you can order directly from their website. In addition to retail outlets, the company's health practitioner program, headed by Dr. Norman Deitch, D.C., provides Penta-Hydrate™ to more than 350 medical doctors, nutritionists, chiropractors and other health care professionals across the U.S.

Uni Key Health Systems, Inc.
P.O. Box 2287
Hayden, ID 83835

orders (800) 888-4353
cust. svc (208) 762-6833
www.unikeyhealth.com

The Verma & Para Systems, as well as the Super GI Cleanse, are recommended in Ann Louise Gittleman's revised and updated Guess What Came to Dinner.

"Water Cure" Products
F. Batmanghelidj, MD
Global Health Solutions
P.O. Box 3189
Falls Church, VA 22043

(703) 848-2333
fax (703) 848-2334
www.watercure.com
Visa/MasterCard orders only:
(800) 759-3999

Dr. Batmanghelidj has many audiotapes and reports on the subject of the importance of water in the human body.

Thermography

William C. Amalu, DC, DABCT, DIACT, FIACT
621 Middlefield Rd.   (650) 361-8908
Redwood City, CA 94063   www.breastthermography.com

If you do not live in the San Francisco Bay Area, Dr. Amalu will be happy to provide a referral to someone in your area who provides thermography.

SUGGESTED READING IN HERBAL MEDICINE

I highly recommend these books to learn more about how nature's pharmacy can share its gifts with your body. Herbal medicine is fascinating. I bet you won't be able to put them down. These books are not listed in order of preference.

Colon Cleansing—The Best Kept Secret
2nd edition, (1989), and
Colon Cleanse the Easy Way
by Jennifer Weiss & Vena Burnett
P.O. Box 5512
Auburn, CA 95604

The Cure for All Diseases
by Hulda Regehr Clark, Ph.D., ND
ProMotion Publishing (1995)
3368 Governor Drive, Suite #144
San Diego, CA 92122

The Herb Lady's Notebook (4th edition)
by Venus Andrecht, ID
Ransom Hill Press (1986)
P.O. Box 325
Ramona, CA 92065
(800) 423-0620
This book can be difficult to come by in regular bookstores. Some health food stores carry it—you will just have to check. You can always order directly from the publisher listed above. If you liked the three stories Ms. Andrecht allowed me to use in this book the rest of her book will tickle your funny bone.

Herbally Yours (3rd edition)
by Penny C. Royal
Sound Nutrition
P.O. Box 55
Hurricane, UT 84737

The How To Herb Book
by Velma J. Keith and Monteen Gordon
Mayfield Publications (1984)
P.O. Box 157
Pleasant Grove, UT 84062

The Little Herb Encyclopedia
by Jack Ritchason
BiWorld Publishers (1982)
Orem, UT

Nutritional Herbology I & II (revised)
by Mark Pedersen
Pedersen Publishing
P.O. Box 761
Bountiful, UT 84010

Own Your Own Body: Herbal Remedies II (revised)
by Dr. Stan Malstrom
BiWorld Publishers (1975)

The Scientific Validation of Herbal Medicine
by Daniel B. Mowrey, Ph.D.
Cormorant Books (1986)

Today's Herbal Health (5th edition)
by Louise Tenny
Woodland Health Books
P.O. Box 1422
Provo, UT

References

1997–2000 Index Medicus — ACA, NEJM, JNCI, J Breast.

1980–1986 Index Medicus — Cancer, AJOG, Thermology.

1996 Text — Atlas of Mammography; New Early Signs in Breast Cancer.

1982 Text — Biomedical Thermology

Aihara, Herman. *Acid & Alkaline.* George Ohsawa Macrobiotic Foundation.

Anderson, Ross, ND. *Are You Clear of Parasites?* 1996.

Balch, James F., MD, and Phyllis A., CNC. *Prescription for Nutritional Healing.* Avery Publishing.

F. Batmanghelidj, M.D, *Your Body's Many Cries for Water*

Brawer, Arthur E., MD. *Holistic Harmony — A Guide to Choosing a Competent Alternative Medicine Provider.*

Burroughs, Stanley. *The Master Cleanser.* 1993.

Cabot, Sandra, MD. *The Liver Cleansing Diet.* 1996.

Cancer Control Journal: A Reference Source Handbook. Vol. 6, No. 7–12.

Cheibner, Viera, Ph.D. *Vaccinations: 100 years of Orthodox Research, and Dangers and Ineffectiveness of Vaccinations* (video). New Atlantean Books.

Chessman, Millan. *Stay Young and Healthy — Through Internal Cleansing.* Vigil Ventures, 1995.

Clark, Hulda, Ph.D., ND. *The Cure for All Cancers.* 1993.

Clark, Hulda, Ph.D., ND. *The Cure for All Diseases.* 1995.

The Colon Health Handbook. Rockridge Publishing Co.

Coulter, Harris L. and Barbara Lowe-Fisher. *A Shot in the Dark.*

Diamond, Harvey and Marilyn. *Fit for Life.*

Diamond, John W., MD, and W. Lee Cowden, MD. *An Alternative Medicine Definitive Guide to Cancer.* Future Medicine Publishing, Inc., 1997.

Epstein, Samuel, MD. *The Politics of Cancer Revisited.* 1998.

Epstein, Samuel, MD, et al. *The Safe Shoppers Bible.* 1995.

Gaeddert, Andrew. *Healing Digestive Disorders.* 1998.

Gittleman, Ann Louise. *Guess What Came to Dinner.* 2001 (revised edition).

Haas, Elson, MD. *The Detox Diet.* 1996.

Haas, Elson, MD. *The False Fat Diet.* 1999.

Haas, Elson, MD. *Staying Healthy With Nutrition.* 1992.

Haas, Elson, MD. *Staying Healthy With the Seasons.* 1981.

Haas, Elson, MD. *The Staying Healthy Shoppers Guide.* 1999.

Hay, Louise. *Heal Your Body.* 1988.

Healthview Newsletter, Issue #1, July 1983.

Howell, Edward. *Enzyme Nutrition: The Food Enzyme Concept.*

Irons, V. Earl. *The Destruction of Your Own Natural Protective Mechanism.* 1995.

Jenks, Jim. *The Eyes Have It.*

Jenks, Jim. *Think and Be Healthy.* 1988.

Jensen, Bernard, DC, ND, Ph.D. *Doctor-Patient Handbook* (10th printing). 1995.

Jensen, Bernard, DC, ND, Ph.D. *Iridology: in the Healing Arts.* Vol. 2, 1982.

Jensen, Bernard, DC, ND, Ph.D. *Iridology Simplified.*

Jensen, Bernard, DC, Ph.D. *Reference to the World Report of Iridology.* Fellowship Journal, December 1974.

Jensen, Bernard, DC, ND, Ph.D. *The Science and Practice of Iridology* (14th printing). 1985.

Jensen, Bernard DC, Ph.D. *Tissue Cleansing Through Bowel Management* (12th edition). 1981.

Kamen, Betty and Si. *Kids Are What They Eat.* Arco Publishing, Inc., 1983.

Kautchakoff, Paul, MD. *The Influence of Food Cooking on the Blood Chemistry of Man.* Institute of Clinical Chemistry, Lausanne, Switzerland, 1930.

Keith, Velma J. and Monteen Gordon. *The How to Herb Book.* Mayfield Publications, 1984.

Kroeger, Hanna. *The Enemy Within.*

Kruhn, Jacqueline, M.D. & Frances Taylor, MA. *Natural Detoxification a Practical Encyclopedia*

Malstrom, Stan. *Own Your Own Body.*

Mendelsohn, Robert S., MD. *How to Raise a Healthy Child In Spite of Your Doctor.* Ballantine Books, 1984.

Merck Manual, 16th edition. *Medical Terms & Jargon.*

Miller, Neil Z. *Vaccinations: Are They Really Safe and Effective?*

Nature's Sunshine. *pH Balancing Simplified* and *An Introduction to Natural Health.*

New Translation of the Holy Scriptures. 1984.

Page, Linda, ND. Ph.D. *Detoxification.* Healthy Healing Publications, 1999.

Page, Linda, ND, Ph.D. *Healthy Healing: An Alternative Healing Reference* (ninth edition). Healthy Healing Publications, 1992.

A Reference Handbook. Cancer Control Journal, Vol. 6., No 7–12, 1985.

Salaman, Maureen. *Nutrition: The Cancer Answer.* 1984.

Santillo, Humbart, MH, ND. *Food Enzymes: The Missing Link.*

Saturday Evening Post. April 1982.

Schiller, Jack G., MD. *Childhood Illness.* Day Books, 1982, p. 123.

Scott, Julian S., Ph.D. *Natural Medicine for Children.* Avon Books, New York.

Shelton, Herbert. *Food Combining Made Easy.* 1982.

Simone, Charles, MD. *Cancer & Nutrition.* 1992.

Smith, Lendon, MD. *Feed Your Kids Right.* Bantam Doubleday Dell Publishing Group, Inc., 1979.

Suggestive Messages for Healing. The American Metabolic Institute.

Thomas, John. *Young Again: How to Reverse the Aging Process*

Tilden, John H., MD. *Toxemia Explained.*

Trenev, Natasha. *Probiotics.* 1998.

Truman, Karol Delmonte. *Feelings Buried Alive Never Die.*

Walker, Norman. *Colon Health: The Key to Vibrant Life.*

Weiss, Jennifer and Vena Burnett. *Colon Cleansing: The Best Kept Secret.* 1989.

Weiss, Jennifer and Vena Burnett. *Colon Cleanse the Easy Way.*

Index

About the Author

Loree Taylor Jordan is a leading health expert and the most appropriate person to write this book. Her extensive background in detoxification and natural healing gives her firsthand experiences that she shares humorously in this one-of-a-kind book. She is not afraid to take on embarrassing and underdiscussed bathroom topics with grace and humor.

Ms. Jordan has 17 years of practical and professional experience as a colon hydrotherapist and holistic health expert. She graduated in 1986 from the National Holistic Institute in Berkeley, California, and is an active member of the International Association of Colon Therapy, the National Speakers Association, and Toastmasters.

Ms. Jordan previously hosted a two-hour radio talk show in the San Francisco Bay Area. Her "don't-sugar-coat-it ... tell-it-like-it-is" persona has given Loree almost a shock jock appeal that really makes people take notice. Her radio show as "The Colonic Queen" was very successful and an extension of her kick-butt, no-holds-barred message. She was personally invited by Anthony Robbins to appear as a speaker in his Life Mastery program.

Ms. Jordan has openly shared her own struggle with weight issues. She is currently researching insulin resistance and metabolic imbalances in weight management. A self-professed reformed "dieting maniac," her upcoming book is titled *Fat and Furious: Overcome Your Body's Resistance to Weight Loss Now!*

Ms. Jordan resides in the Bay Area, where she was born. She is an avid animal lover and lives with two dogs and six cats. She is the mother of two grown sons.

Quick Order Form

To order *Detox for Life* books, and for author interviews/speaking engagements, contact LTJ Associates at (408) 379-9488.

Quantity purchases: This book is available at special discounts for gifts, premiums, promotions, educational use, or resale. Contact LTJ Associates.

Fax orders:	(408) 379-1152. Send this form
Telephone orders:	(800) 247-6553. For book and tape orders only. Please have your Visa or MasterCard ready.
E-mail orders:	www.Detoxforlife.net
Postal orders:	Bookmasters, P.O. Box 388, Ashland, OH 44805 (800) 247-6553.

❑ Please send the following books or tapes:

_____

_____

Please send me FREE information about:

❑ upcoming books/tapes   ❑ Loree's products/programs

❑ speaking/seminars   ❑ consulting/health coaching

❑ Please add me to your mailing list.

Name _____

Address _____

City _____ State ____ Zip _____

Telephone (day) _____ (eve) _____

E-mail _____

Sales tax:	Please add 8.25% for products shipped to California.
Shipping:	$4.50 U.S. for the first book and $2 for each additional product. All books are shipped Priority Mail or UPS Ground (please specify).

Payment: ❑ Check   ❑ Visa   ❑ MasterCard

Card number _____

Name on card _____ Exp. _____